PREPARE FOR COMBAT

Strength Training for the Martial Arts

MIKHAIL KRUPNIK,
M.S., NSCA-CPT

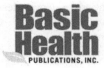

Basic Health
PUBLICATIONS, INC.

The information contained in this book is based upon the research and personal and professional experiences of the author. It is not intended as a substitute for consulting with your physician or other healthcare provider. Any attempt to diagnose and treat an illness should be done under the direction of a healthcare professional.

The publisher does not advocate the use of any particular healthcare protocol but believes the information in this book should be available to the public. The publisher and author are not responsible for any adverse effects or consequences resulting from the use of the suggestions, preparations, or procedures discussed in this book. Should the reader have any questions concerning the appropriateness of any procedures or preparation mentioned, the author and the publisher strongly suggest consulting a professional healthcare advisor.

Basic Health Publications, Inc.
www.basichealthpub.com

Library of Congress Cataloging-in-Publication Data

Krupnik, Mikhail
    Prepare for combat : weight training for the martial arts / Mikhail Krupnik.
        p. cm.
    Includes bibliographical references and index.

    ISBN-13: 978-1-59120-183-0 (Pbk.)
    ISBN-13: 978-1-68162-771-7 (Hardcover)

    1. Martial arts--Training. 2. Weight training. I. Title.

GV1102.7.T7K78   2006
613.7'148—dc22

                                    2006019267

Editor: Carol Rosenberg • Illustrations: Alan Pastrana
Typesetting/Layout: Gary A. Rosenberg • Cover design: Mike Stromberg

Contents

To my family and friends for providing me with
their continued support and understanding,
which has made my work and this book possible.

Foreword

As an avid martial arts practitioner, I highly recommend Mikhail Krupnik's book *Prepare for Combat,* as it will serve as a very valuable tool for all martial artists. As a former professional welterweight kickboxer, I could only have wished to have such a resource at my fingertips during my competitive career, before a shoulder injury had forced me to the sidelines of professional fighting.

I first met Mikhail Krupnik when he and I literally bumped into each other at a kickboxing event. We immediately hit it off. That weekend, I read the 1999 edition of *Prepare for Combat,* and the following week I booked a private lesson with him. Mikhail's teachings in the book and in person are equally good and helpful. Reading *Prepare for Combat* is like having a private session with him, where you receive in-depth advice and knowledge suited to your own personal needs.

Mr. Krupnik taught a hands-on seminar at my school, and my students and I still discuss and practice his concepts. I truly believe that *Prepare for Combat* will open up doors for beginners, intermediate, and advanced students alike.

—Shihan Thomas R. Ingargiola
Eighth-Degree Black belt, Shaolin Kempo

Introduction

It was once commonly accepted by the martial arts community that engaging in any form of weight training was detrimental to one's performance of the art. The old school of thought taught us that training with weights would hinder our development of flexibility, speed, and agility. To be effective fighters, we had to be quick and light on our feet like Bruce Lee and other prominent martial artists, all of whom were slim and small, but quite powerful. Their quickness and lightning-fast techniques more than made up for their lack of size and muscle mass.

We were taught that karate is all about good technique and proper timing and that muscle size has little to do with it. After all, the art of self-defense lies in the premise that smaller, weaker people can defend themselves effectively against much larger and stronger opponents. In fact, this is exactly what attracted many of us to the art of self-defense: the desire to learn to defend ourselves, even if we are not that big and strong. While it's true that good technique and proper timing are essential, there's no valid reason to think that building muscle will hinder a person's effectiveness as a martial artist. In fact, just the opposite is true: the stronger you are, the better able you will be to defend yourself and use your skills as a martial artist in competition.

The argument against weight training for the benefit of martial arts was largely based on tradition and popular sentiment, not on facts. Fortunately, over the past few decades, the attitude toward weight training has changed—largely due to an abundance of scientific data showing the positive effects of weight training for all kinds of sports. We, as a society, no longer view someone who trains with weights as a mindless bodybuilder, whose only priority in life is to build bigger muscles. Modern-day athletes have much to gain by using weights to improve performance in their chosen sport. As practitioners of the martial arts, we are no different from other dedicated athletes and should therefore consider the potential benefits of weight training in our sport. These benefits include increased strength, increased resistance to fatigue, and decreased risk of injury.

Nevertheless, the stigma of weight training was once so pervasive across the karate community that some traditionalists still refuse to let go of this misconception. They believe that the strength gains are not specific to the demands of karate and that the benefits derived from these gains are outweighed by the perceived loss of speed and flexibility. Although you could slow yourself down by taking bodybuilding to the extreme, a well-designed, sport-specific weight-training routine—in addition to your regular martial arts practice—will make you stronger, not slower. In some cases, it can even improve your speed.

In *Prepare for Combat*, you'll learn how to design a weight-training program to fit your individual needs and goals. From all-important safety issues, determining your level of fitness, and setting your goals, to specific exercises, sample routines, and even proper nutrition—this book covers everything you need to know to enhance your performance as a martial artist with weight training.

CHAPTER 1

Weight Training
and the Martial Artist

ith a well-designed weight-training program, you can expect a significant increase in the strength of your muscles with only a minimal increase in muscle mass in as few as thirty minutes a day, two to three times a week. The gains in muscle mass—even if they are relatively significant—will not interfere with your speed. This is because as your weight increases, so will your body's ability to handle the weight. As long as you continue to train and practice your martial art regularly, you will be as quick as you always were. And, as far as your flexibility is concerned, you'll remain limber as long as you don't neglect your regular stretching regimen. Rest assured, there's just no scientific evidence to suggest that weight training will make you slower or less flexible due to the increase in muscle mass. In the final analysis, as long as you continue to train and perform martial-arts specific techniques and as long as you stretch on a regular basis, you will be as flexible and as quick as you were before you started your weight-training program. Adding weight training to your routine will simply improve your conditioning and your overall performance in the martial arts.

In this chapter, we'll take a look at what you can expect from weight training, important safety considerations, and the eight principles of weight training that you should keep in mind when developing your program.

WHAT YOU CAN EXPECT FROM WEIGHT TRAINING

No matter what style of martial arts you practice and no matter your age, gender, body type, or level of fitness, you *can* benefit from a well-designed, realistic weight-training program. Obviously, the most important benefit of weight training is an increase in muscular strength. This increase in strength is the result of two phenomena. The first is improved neuromuscular adaptation—the ability of a specific muscle group to recall and utilize a larger percentage of available muscle fibers. This perceived increase in strength during the first stages of weight training (approximately one month) is largely due to improved efficiency rather than an increase in muscle size. The second, and more significant, phenomenon is an increase in muscle size, resulting in increased strength. Also, as your overall muscle size increases, your body will be able to utilize even more muscle fibers from the larger supply of muscle mass. This increase in strength leads to improved striking power, more effective blocks, stronger stances, improved agility, and increased resistance to fatigue and injury.

Let's examine each of these benefits.

Improved Striking Power

There are two ways to increase the effectiveness of your attack: 1) by increasing the velocity, or speed, of your strikes, and 2) by increasing the weight, or mass, behind your strikes. Although weight training doesn't guarantee an increase in speed, it will certainly allow you to generate much more power. If you maintain your speed through proper training as you increase your strength, your punching and kicking techniques will be significantly more powerful.

More Effective Blocking Techniques

When it comes to blocking an attack, proper timing and speed are, of course, essential. You should certainly strive for both. However, you can make your blocks even more effective by also increasing the power behind them. As your strength increases, you will be able to block an incoming punch or kick more effectively, even if you don't have the perfect timing in that particular instance. While it's true that doesn't make it a better block, it does allow you to compensate for lack of good technique, if necessary. If you can combine perfect timing and added strength, you will be a much more formidable competitor.

Stronger Stances and Improved Agility

Strengthening the muscles in your lower body with weight-training exercises targeted to key areas will improve your balance and provide you with more overall stability. With better balance and a more stable base, your opponents will have a greater difficultly trying to sweep you, knock you down, or even buckle your stance. A stronger foundation will give you more leverage during kicking and punching and more stability for better blocking. Moreover, a stronger lower body will improve your ability to move with ease. This will result in faster and more explosive attacks as well as a better reaction time for more effective counterattacks.

Decreased Risk of Injury

Injury prevention is one of the major benefits of weight training. One way in which weight training can protect you against injury is by increasing your lean body mass. What this means is that muscle increases in mass, bone increases in density, and tendons and ligaments increase in strength. As a result, your bones and joints become fortified and less susceptible to injury.

The second way in which weight training can reduce the risk of injury is by building up the muscles that are not being developed during the course of karate training. Martial arts training tends to overdevelop some muscle groups, primarily pectorals (chest muscles), abdominal (stomach or oblique muscles), and hip flexors (the knee-raising muscles), and it neglects some opposing muscle groups, primarily upper- and lower-back muscles. As a result, the overdeveloped muscles become stronger and tighter at the expense of opposing, underdeveloped muscle groups, which become weaker and less resilient. This offsets your posture and puts more pressure on the shoulder, hip, and knee joints. If left unresolved, this postural imbalance could lead to acute lower back, knee, and/or shoulder injuries, which can become chronic if left untreated. To correct your posture, you would simply need to stretch the overdeveloped muscles and build up the underdeveloped muscles with a well-balanced weight-training and stretching program. This means strengthening your back muscles, especially your lower back, by performing pull-ups, seated rows, and back extensions, and stretching your overused hip flexor and chest muscles.

Weight training also helps to speed up the healing process when an injury is sustained. This is a direct result of the increase in muscle mass and the consequent increase in circulation, which raises the supply of the necessary nutrients to help repair the damaged area. (See the inset "Injured?" below for important information.)

Increased Resistance to Fatigue

Weaker muscles are more prone to fatigue whereas stronger muscles are more durable. Increasing muscular strength and/or endurance will improve your stamina in competition and in training. Better stamina allows a fighter to last longer and maintain good form and sharp technique in the process. This is the variable that usually separates the winners from the losers during the later rounds of competition. If winning is important to you, you have your work cut out for you.

SAFETY CONSIDERATIONS

The best weight-training program is the one that will allow you to achieve your objective of improving muscular strength and/or muscular endurance and ultimately improve your performance in the martial arts. To achieve your objective, your weight-training program needs to be safe above all else. If you keep getting injured during training, it will be very difficult for you to be consistent. If you are not consistent, it is almost impossible to get better. To stay consistent and injury-free, some safety principles have to be implemented in your program. These include determining safety of participation, mastering the proper form, spotting, appropriate exercise attire, and proper warm-up and cool-down periods.

Injured?

If you become injured, be sure to consult your doctor or a physical therapist to find out just how serious the injury is and how much time you'll need to recover from this setback. Make sure you allow for a sufficient amount of time to pass before you resume your training as before. If you try to come back too soon before you fully recover from your injury, you may reinjure yourself which can result in a chronic problem. At that point, no amount of weight training can help you.

Determining Safety of Participation

To avoid any serious complications, it is necessary to know if you have any limitations to exercise. Make sure you know what your limitations are before you begin training. In general, heavy resistance training is not recommended for:

- People with a documented history of heart disease.
- People with high blood pressure.
- People who have, or have had, serious back or other joint injuries.
- People who are extremely overweight (50 pounds over ideal body weight).
- Children under the age of sixteen (without a physician's approval and parental consent).

Mastering the Form

It is very important to learn the proper weight-lifting technique before you move on to heavier weights and fewer repetitions. It is easier to master the form if you are not struggling to lift the weight. That is one of the reasons why I recommend lifting lighter weights and performing a higher number of repetitions when you first start your weight-training program. If you are not sure about how much weight you can handle, select the least level of resistance, especially if you are still learning the proper form. It is better to do more repetitions with less weight and do the exercise properly than it is to struggle to lift more weight and risk a chance of injury.

Regardless of the exercise, make sure you are familiar with the equipment you have selected. Know the function of each machine or exercise station you are training on. Know how to adjust each machine to your own size, and know how to set the right resistance. Before beginning your set, make sure you have enough room and that no one is in your way. Assume a stable position and make sure to have a firm grip on the bar or handle. Each repetition should be executed in one single fluid motion through a full range of motion. You should take 3–5 seconds executing each repetition, remembering to inhale at the start of each repetition and to exhale throughout the work phase. Even if you are experienced at weight training, you should spend one day a week perfecting your technique by working with a lighter weight than usual and performing more repetitions.

Spotting

Consider recruiting a partner to exercise with. There are two reasons why this is a good idea. The primary reason is safety; the other is motivation.

Your partner can spot you when necessary to help you avoid accidents. He or she can assist you with your last repetition or help you get out of trouble if you cramp up or temporarily lose your concentration. Your spotter can also watch your form to make sure you are lifting properly. (If a mirror is available, you can watch your own form.)

If you are training on machines, it's not as important to have a partner spot you. However, if you are using free-weights, exercising without someone to spot you is like riding a motorcycle without a helmet. It can be done, but it's not recommended. If you are weight training without a partner at a local gym, you will rarely be turned down if you ask a fellow member to spot you. You can always return the favor.

A partner can also motivate you to work harder or to take it easy when necessary. The bottom line is, it is more effective and more fun to train with someone who shares your interests.

Appropriate Exercise Attire and Other Accessories

It is not necessary to spend a lot of money on your workout attire. All you need is a pair of good-quality cross-trainers, tennis, or basketball shoes; a pair of cotton shorts and a cotton t-shirt to stay cool and comfortable while you exercise; a pair of weight-lifting gloves for a better grip; and a weight belt for extra lower-back support.

Proper Warm-Up/Cool-down Periods

It is important to warm up your muscles before you begin your weight-training session to make them more receptive to the new level of stress. The warm-up phase should not last longer than 20 minutes, and should include 5–10 minutes of a low-intensity exercise such as jumping rope, jogging in place, or doing jumping jacks. This should be followed by 10 minutes of stretching. You could also include a low-weight, high-repetition set before your main workout for each exercise you plan to perform. This will allow you to perfect your form for lifting before you work with heavier weights.

The cool-down portion of your routine should include some basic upper- and lower-body stretching exercises to help reduce the soreness associated with resistance training. While recommended stretches are not included in this book, you should already be familiar with a variety of stretches from training in the martial arts. If not, I suggest you seek out a good resource on flexibility training.

THE EIGHT PRINCIPLES OF WEIGHT TRAINING

To improve muscle strength and/or muscle endurance, there are several exercise principles you need to apply to your weight-training program. The following eight principles are essential for achieving success: 1) Mode of Exercise, 2) Intensity/Muscle Overload, 3) Duration, 4) Recovery, 5) Consistency/Frequency, 6) Progression/Steady Progress, 7) Specificity, and 8) Sequence. Let's take a look at each of these.

PRINCIPLE # 1—MODE OF EXERCISE

The mode of exercise refers to the type of activity you choose to perform to help increase your strength or endurance in the specific area of the body—for example, performing lunges or squats for improving lower-body strength or endurance.

PRINCIPLE #2—INTENSITY/MUSCLE OVERLOAD

In order for your muscles to get stronger, they need to be exposed to higher than usual levels of stress. Select an amount of weight you can lift at least 5 times but not more than 20. This means starting with 65–85 percent of your maximum capacity, or one-repetition maximum (1RM). (To determine your 1RM, see Appendix A.)

PRINCIPLE #3—DURATION

The total number of repetitions, sets, and exercises performed will determine the length of your workout. The total time spent in the weight room, including recovery time between sets, should not exceed one hour (see Principle #4 below).

For maximum results, you have to perform as many repetitions as you can with the resistance level chosen to reach temporary muscle failure (5–20 reps). If the weight you pick is consistently too light, you will not reach temporary muscle failure and will not achieve a significant increase in your strength or endurance over time.

The number of repetitions will be determined by the amount of weight you select. The heavier the weight, the fewer repetitions you will be able to perform. Regardless of the number of repetitions you will be able to execute, once you've reached the point of muscle failure, you've completed one set. The number of sets should be 1–4 sets per exercise. The num-

> **Repetition (rep)**—A single execution of exercise; for example, one single squat or one pull-up.
>
> **Set**—A number of repetitions completed in succession; for example, 10 squats per set.

ber of exercises should be 1–3 per body part. The total number of sets you perform will depend on the number of exercises you would like to complete, your level of fitness, and the amount of time you have to train. Approximately 10–20 sets per workout will suffice.

PRINCIPLE # 4—RECOVERY

There are three types of recovery: 1) the recovery time between sets of the same exercise, 2) the recovery time between different exercises, and 3) the recovery time between workouts of the same muscle groups.

If you are performing multiple sets of the same exercise or targeting the same muscle group with different exercises, the recovery time between sets is 2–4 minutes. For example, wait 2–4 minutes between pull-ups and pull-downs since these exercises target the same muscle group.

The recovery time between different exercises targeting different muscle groups is 30 seconds to 2 minutes. For example, wait 30 seconds to 2 minutes between seated rows and squats, which target different body parts.

The recovery time between workouts targeting the *same muscle groups* should be 48 hours. For example, if you exercise your chest muscles on Monday, wait until Wednesday to exercise that body part again. If you still feel sore on Wednesday, rest for another day. If it takes longer than that to recover, you have overtrained (see page 19 for more information on overtraining).

PRINCIPLE #5—CONSISTENCY/FREQUENCY

Being consistent is the key to success in any program. You must lift weights at least 2–3 times a week to see significant gains in muscular strength or endurance.

PRINCIPLE #6—PROGRESSION/STEADY PROGRESS

As you continue to advance in your weight-training program, you will experience an increase in your muscular strength and/or muscular endurance level. You will notice that you are able to do more reps with the same amount of weight. As you get stronger, it is important to continue to challenge yourself by periodically increasing the weight you are using to train. Retest yourself every few weeks. If you notice an improvement, use this new maximum level to select your training weight.

PRINCIPLE # 7—SPECIFICITY

Weight training is very specific. You can only strengthen the muscles you specifically target for improvement. This means that all major muscle groups must be exercised during the course of your weekly training program if you want to get stronger all around. Exercising only some muscle groups will not improve those that are not being used. It is also recommended that you vary your routine to work on muscular strength some days and muscular endurance on others. If you emphasize only one of these components, you will do little to improve the other.

PRINCIPLE #8—SEQUENCE

Sequence refers to the order in which you proceed with your exercise routine. To get the most out of your workout, begin with multi-joint exercises such as the squat, pull-up, or chest press, and work your way down to single-joint isolation exercises, such as heel raise, biceps curl, and triceps extension.

Multi-joint exercises involve more than one joint at the same time and are more demanding because they recruit a larger percentage of total muscle mass than single-joint exercises. Always start your workout with the most difficult exercises because that is when you are most alert and energized. This maximizes productivity and reduces the risk of injury.

CONCLUSION

Weight training is one of the safest and most effective forms of exercise. For someone who participates in the martial arts, as well as other sports, weight training provides another dimension to your overall development. It has been shown that a number of injuries can occur from repetitive stress. Weight training allows you to maintain your level of fitness and develop other areas of fitness while receiving a break from the repetitive stress of martial arts training. As long as you adhere to the basic principles outlined in this chapter, you will increase your overall strength and endurance and elevate your performance in the martial arts to new heights.

CHAPTER 2

The Right Weight-Training Program for You

When designing your program, be sure to keep in mind that everyone is different. We all have different abilities, time constraints, obligations, and goals. What's right for one person might not be right for another and in some cases, can even be detrimental. So, before designing your weight-training program, you should determine your level of fitness— your strengths and weaknesses, as well as your limitations. Then, determine your immediate and long-term goals. That's where this chapter comes in. It will help you assess your overall fitness level and get you on track to help you set some realistic and measurable goals. Let's take a look at the steps you should take to design the most appropriate program for your needs.

DETERMINING YOUR FITNESS LEVEL

To ensure a safe and effective program, you need to establish a starting point. This means you must rank yourself on the basis of your knowledge, experience, and level of fitness. Ask yourself, "How much experience with weight training have I had?" Be honest. Even if you have used weights in training in the past but have not been training for a while, do not be quick to rank yourself as an advanced student and attempt to train as such. It is better to underestimate your capabilities in the beginning than risk injuring yourself.

In general, if you have been weight training for fewer than six months, you can call yourself a beginner in weight training, even if you are a black belt in your martial art. Keep in mind that training is very specific. Being an expert in one area of training does not make you an expert in another. People with limited knowledge and experience with weight training should not assume they know more than they actually do. Be realistic about your abilities, and you will be much more successful with your program.

Those who have six months to two years experience can be considered beginner to intermediate level students, assuming they have been training consistently—that is, two to three times per week and good, reliable information about weight training was available. If you have been weight training consistently for longer than two years, you may consider yourself an advanced student. You should remember, however, that even experts have room for improvement.

Depending on your level of experience and knowledge, choose the routine that is right for you. For example, beginners will start at the base-training stage. Intermediate students will start at the base-training, intermediate, or advanced stage. Advanced students will start at the advanced, maintenance, or recovery stage. (See Chapter 3 for an explanation of these stages.) For now, the important thing is to know which stage of development you are in and which weight-training program is the safest and most effective for you to start with. Remember that if you are in doubt, start at the beginning.

The next step is to determine your present level of fitness. You need to find out how strong you are before you can start training. For example, how many push-ups or pull-ups can you do in succession? Can you squat or bench-press the equivalent of your own body weight? This can be accomplished by determining your current level of muscular strength and/or muscular endurance using several different exercise stations. (See Appendix A for testing procedures.)

If you have access to and experience with weight-training equipment, you can start with your lower-body strength testing by performing one-repetition maximum (1RM) squat and/or leg press or leg extension and leg curl. For upper-body strength testing, the best exercises are 1RM on the bench press, pull-downs, seated rows, and overhead presses. Determining the maximum amount of weight you can lift one time, your 1RM, on as many of these exercise stations as possible will give you a better idea of your overall level of strength. You can also add several muscular endurance tests such as maximum pull-ups, maximum push-ups, and one-minute sit-ups to round off the testing procedure. It is important to have a spotter assist you while you are performing these tests. This will not only allow you to give your maximum effort, but also will help prevent any possible mishaps.

If you are not very experienced with weight training or you do not have someone to spot you, use the same exercise equipment to determine the maximum amount of resistance or weight you are able to lift or move ten times—ten-repetition maximum (10RM). This is a safer alternative to 1RM. You can also perform the following: maximum push-up test, one-minute sit-up test, and maximum pull-up test. When selecting the resistance level to train with, you can use the 10RM level as your starting weight. (Once again, for more details about the testing procedures, see Appendix A.)

There are two reasons why it's important to establish your maximum capacity before beginning your program: 1) it will be easier to select the proper amount of weight to work with, and 2) it will be easier to gauge your progress with retesting. Once you have established your initial level of muscular strength and/or muscular endurance by performing the tests in Appendix A, you can use these results to set new goals and the proper course of action.

If you are starting a weight-training program for the first time or if you are coming back from a long layoff, don't try to do too much. Limit yourself to several tests just so you have some idea of your level of fitness.

ESTABLISHING YOUR OBJECTIVES

The more specific you are in formulating your objectives, the better chance you have of designing and sticking with the right program and achieving your goals. Your objectives might change over the course of the year. Try to stick to one or two different objectives per cycle (six months to one year). If you change your goals every other week, you won't be able to accomplish anything. Once you decide what you want to accomplish with your weight-training program, allow yourself enough time to achieve your objective before moving on to the next one. Your training program will depend on your objectives, your time, and your equipment availability. Appendix B contains a questionnaire that will help you set the right course of action. Do not be discouraged if you don't have the luxury of a lot of time or a fitness-club membership. As long as you have the desire, you can create an effective and safe program with a minimal amount of time and equipment. It is, however, easier if you are not limited by these two variables.

How do you determine which weight-training program is right for you? Well, if you are a beginner, you don't have much choice in the matter. You'll need to stick with muscular-endurance training for the first several months using a limited number of sets, paying extra attention to proper form, and allowing yourself enough time to recover. The goals for the first couple of months should be to build a base and to learn how to exercise in a safe and effective manner. Once you have a base and some experience, you'll have to decide which component of your martial art you need to focus on the most. The following is a list of potential problems regularly encountered by martial art students and some of the possible weight-training solutions.

PROBLEM: Weak and/or ineffective punching or blocking techniques.

SOLUTION: Emphasize building strength in your upper body. Perform as many upper-body exercises as possible during the course of the week, emphasizing heavier weight, fewer repetitions, and longer rest periods. (Regardless of the ultimate objective, beginners need to start with muscular-endurance training and eventually build up to strength training.)

PROBLEM: Weak and/or ineffective kicking techniques.

SOLUTION: Emphasize building strength in your lower body. Perform as many lower-body exercises as possible during the course of the week, emphasizing heavier weight, fewer repetitions, and longer rest periods. (Regardless of the ultimate objective, beginners need to start with muscular-endurance training and eventually build up to strength training.)

PROBLEM: Inability to sustain the same intensity in the later rounds of competition and/or training.

SOLUTION: Emphasize muscular-endurance training, but also include some strength training during the course of the week or during the same workout. Weight train after your main martial arts workout when you are tired, but not if you are exhausted. If you are exhausted, you will be more susceptible to injury. Make sure to allow extra recovery time the following day—in other words, take the day off.

PROBLEM: Frequent overuse injuries.

SOLUTION: Muscular-endurance training that emphasizes the muscles around the troubled joint will help solve this problem. For example, to effectively compensate for a weak knee joint, you'll need to build up your gluteus (buttock muscles), quads (front of the thigh), hamstrings (back of the thigh), calf, and lower and upper back muscles.

If you suffer from frequent overuse injuries, weight training should be done before your martial arts training to minimize the risk of injury. You can also weight train on your easier or less-intense martial arts training days but never in place of your planned rest day.

PROBLEM: Little time available during the day.

SOLUTION: If you have a limited amount of time to train, you can do one of two things. 1) You can limit the number of sets per workout to 1–2 sets, keeping the intensity and number of exercises the same, or 2) you can limit the number of exercises per workout to 3–5 exercises, keeping the intensity and number of sets the same.

You can also limit the number of sets and the number of exercises to a recommended minimum, based on the stage of development and your fitness level, while maintaining the same intensity. If you have a lot of experience with weight training, you can even reduce the amount of rest between sets or do "supersets"—combining two or three different exercises into one set.

Use your time wisely by performing multi-joint exercises such as pull-downs and leg presses, and reducing the number of single-joint isolation exercises such as arm curls and triceps presses.

WEIGHT TRAINING WITHOUT WEIGHING YOURSELF DOWN

To get the most out of your weight-training program without interfering with your martial arts training, always schedule your workouts around your karate classes and certainly not instead of them. After all, if you are weight training to improve your martial arts performance, it doesn't make sense to spend so much time and energy that you have nothing left for your martial arts training. Under no circumstances should you ever expend your energy lifting weights prior to learning or perfecting an important move or technique. Your muscles will be too tired and less likely to remember the correct execution.

It's ideal to schedule your weight-training workout a day prior to or a day after your karate class. When you must do both on the same day, be sure the following day is a day of rest or at least a very light workout. Weight training is a very strenuous activity, and your body will require

Training to Improve Muscle Strength and/or Endurance

In general, there are two components you can improve with resistance training: one is muscular strength, and the other is muscular endurance. Knowing when to do one or the other is part of the art of weight training.

Muscle strength is the ability of the muscle to generate maximum force for one single repetition. This component of fitness is measured by a one-repetition maximum (1RM) or any maximum effort test—for example, the most amount of weight a person can lift one time or the maximum force of a single kick or punch. To improve your strength, select heavy resistance, 80–90 percent of your 1RM, and perform fewer repetitions (5–10 reps).

Muscle endurance is the ability to repeat a muscle contraction against submaximal resistance for a prolonged period of time—for example, the ability to kick, punch, and/or block repeatedly with less than maximum effort for a few seconds. To improve your muscular endurance, select lower resistance, 65–80 percent of your 1RM, and perform a greater number of repetitions (10–20 reps).

It is very important to develop both strength and endurance for the purpose of martial arts training. If you have a strong block/punch/kick combination, you can end a fight quickly. But if you need to fight or compete for more than a few seconds, you have to be able to do so without tiring. Both of these variables can be improved with resistance training. As described above, the difference is in the amount of weight you are lifting and the number of reps and sets you accomplish.

The level of resistance determines the number of repetitions you can complete. The more weight you pile up, the fewer repetitions you will be able to do. In either case, do as many repetitions as possible with the resistance you select. Do not get caught up in numbers—the key is that you perform each repetition with perfect form. It is the total amount of time the muscle group is stressed, not the number of repetitions that is most important.

more time to recover from your workouts if you do both on the same day. This means you'll need to take at least one day off each week—no karate training or weight training—to fully recover. If necessary, take an additional day off from weight training to recover, especially if you are a beginner. Keep in mind that your body will get stronger during rest periods as it tries to recover and repair itself after a bout of exercise.

You must keep in mind that rest is a crucial part of your exercise program. The harder you train, the longer your recovery period should be. Resting allows your body to recuperate and adapt to the new level of stress. In the process, your body gets stronger. With time, this increase in strength allows you to increase the level of resistance.

If you do not allow your body sufficient time to recuperate, it will not be able to handle as much stress the next time you train. If you continue to exert yourself without resting—in other words, if you overtrain—you will not notice any improvements, and eventually experience a significant drop in your performance due to physical fatigue. This does not have to happen. You simply need to recognize some of the signs of overtraining and stop all training until your body fully recovers. The following section discusses some of the early signs of overtraining.

How to Recognize When You're Overtraining

Become familiar with the following signs of overtraining so you can make the necessary changes to your routine to ensure that you are getting the most benefit from your program.

- **Prolonged muscle soreness**—Some muscle soreness is to be expected, especially during the initial stage of a weight-training program. However, after the first few weeks of training, any soreness that you will experience should subside after one or two days of rest. If you are still sore after that time has passed, you've overdone it.

- **Elevated resting heart rate**—An increase in your resting heart rate of ten beats per minute or more is a sign of too much physical and/or mental stress. To check your resting heart rate, perform the following test as soon as you wake up in the morning: sit up and place your three middle fingers on your opposite wrist. Using a stopwatch or secondhand on a clock, count the number of beats for six seconds. Multiply the number by ten. This is your one-minute resting heart rate. Perform this test periodically. If the number increases, it may be a sign that you're overtraining.

- **Loss of appetite**—If you are training regularly, your appetite should be greater than normal. If your appetite diminishes, it could mean too much work and not enough rest. Loss of appetite usually leads to a significant decrease in body weight and a subsequent drop in performance.

- **Significant drop in performance**—An inability to complete a scheduled workout—that is, not being able to handle the usual amount of weight, sets, reps, or exercises—or the inability to perform up to your potential during competition or training are signs of overtraining.

- **Decreased resistance to illness or injury**—As the total exercise load increases, your body gets stronger and is able to withstand more stress. However, if you increase the level of stress too much or too soon, you can reach the point of diminishing returns. When the amount of stress reaches that point, the extra demand can actually weaken your system and reduce your body's ability to endure and fight off illness. As a result, you become more susceptible to nagging injuries and common infections.
- **Insomnia**—The inability to sleep at night due to restlessness is a telltale sign of overtraining.

Other symptoms of overtraining include an inability to concentrate and be productive in general, lack of motivation, irritability, and low sex drive.

If you experience more than one of these symptoms for more than three days, modify your exercise program or simply add another rest day. Do not ignore the signs of overtraining. If you consistently ignore these important signs, you are risking burnout or a more serious injury.

Recovery Guidelines

While it's a good idea to recognize the signs of overtraining, it's an even better idea not to over train in the first place. The following recovery guidelines should help.

- **Get enough sleep**—Nighttime rest is the easiest and most natural way for your body to recover. In addition to scheduling regular rest days, you must get enough sleep during the night (8–9 hours) to feel well rested. If you are not lucky enough to get the required amount of sleep, try scheduling regular naps during the day. The effects of sleeplessness are cumulative. This means that if you sleep one hour less per day, in a week you will be seven hours behind. At that point, to catch up you would need to sleep seven extra hours on weekends. If you do not catch up on your sleep, you will feel chronically fatigued.
- **Allow enough time to recover**—If you are not sure whether or not you have recovered from a bout of exercise, it is better to take another day off. The fresher you feel, the more productive you will be when you

train. As you'll learn in Chapter 3, it's a good idea to schedule at least one full day of complete rest every week and one recovery week every couple of months. Also, consider taking 2–3 weeks off from training each year after completing a cycle.

- **Increase your training load gradually**—Do not be in a hurry to improve. The total amount of the training load should be increased in a slow and consistent manner. Start with the least amount of work required based on your test results (see Appendix A). When you feel you are ready to progress to the next level, do not try to increase all of the elements of your program at once. Instead, increase only one element at a time. For example, you can increase the total number of sets per workout every other week. Or you can increase the resistance level for 2–3 exercises at a time while keeping the number of sets the same. Your body requires at least 1–2 weeks of training to adapt each time you advance to a new level of work. When you are ready to increase the resistance level of your workout, keep the number of sets and the number of exercises constant. If you decide to increase the number of sets or exercises, keep the intensity constant.

- **Get enough fuel**—You must eat enough to sustain your daily amount of exercise. If you are constantly low on energy, you cannot perform to your full potential. This will impede your progress. (See Chapter 6 for some helpful nutritional guidelines.)

- **Stay well hydrated**—You must consume enough fluids in the form of water or sports drinks during the day especially in hotter months—six to ten 8-ounce glasses a day. You'll know you are drinking enough if your urine is clear. Lack of fluid consumption can lead to dehydration and significantly reduce your productivity during training and competition.

- **Be aware of the effects of outside stress**—If you are under a lot of mental or physical stress at home or on the job, take it into consideration when you train. This outside stress can affect your workout negatively and cause you to feel sluggish and tired. Sometimes it is better not to train and simply take a day off from exercising to recuperate. If you do decide to train, don't force your body to perform. If you are down for whatever reason, you will not be able to train at the intensity required to improve. So, if you can't be productive, at least try to recuperate for the next time.

- **Make sure you are not sick**—When you come down with a virus or sustain an injury, your body will require lots of energy to fight off the illness or repair the damaged area. Putting more stress on your body by exercising during these times can be counterproductive. Exercise can prolong the effects or symptoms of your sickness or injury and delay your recovery time. Therefore, if you do get sick or injured, be sure to consider taking a few days off until you feel better. You won't lose much headway in one week.

- **Cut down on competition**—Too much competition is very stressful on your body. If you are noticing a drop in your performance, you might need to cut down on the number of tournaments in which you compete during the year. Some downtime allows you to recover mentally as well as physically.

- **Listen to your body**—Always pay close attention to your body, and if possible, monitor your vital signs on a daily basis, including your heart rate, blood pressure, and body weight. If you monitor your vital signs every day, you'll notice changes right away.

  As mentioned previously, one of the first signs of overtraining, or rest deprivation, is a rise in your resting pulse (ten or more beats per minute higher than usual), indicating that you need a day off. A significant rise in your resting blood pressure can also be an indication of too much stress on your body. Weighing yourself every day allows you to monitor your food intake. If you notice a significant weight loss of two pounds or more in a week, increase your daily food and fluid intake to avoid burnout.

CONCLUSION

Designing the right program is as much an art as it is a science. Knowing your body and understanding how the program you follow will affect your overall development and performance is a process that requires patience and determination. No matter how careful and meticulous you are in following your strategy, you will undoubtedly suffer from some setbacks. Don't be afraid to reevaluate, and if necessary, change your program if it is not working for you. You can also ask experts for advice. You can benefit greatly by learning from a wily veteran who has gone through the same process you are presently going through. It is easier and less painful to learn from someone else's mistakes.

CHAPTER 3

The Stages of the Weight-Training Cycle

Your weight-training program needs to have structure for maximum effectiveness. This is easily accomplished by dividing your program into five separate periods, or stages of development—the base-training stage, the intermediate stage, the advanced/strength-building stage, the maintenance stage, and the recovery stage. All of these important stages, which are described in this chapter, need to be followed in their proper order. Skipping or curtailing any of them may lead to injury or overtraining. It is okay to extend the base-training or maintenance stages or even the recovery stage, but it can be dangerous to prolong the advanced stage beyond the recommended period. Later, in Appendix C, you can review and implement the sample weight-training routines for each of these stages.

STAGE 1: BASE-TRAINING STAGE

This is the initial muscular-endurance building stage, characterized by moderate weight and high repetitions.

- **Number of exercises**—No more than 15 exercises per workout, all major muscle groups (full-body workout)
- **Intensity**—60–75 percent 1RM or one level below 10RM
- **Duration**—10–20 reps, 1–3 sets per exercise (start with 1 set and increase to a maximum of 3 sets)
- **Frequency**—3–4 times per week or every other day

- **Recovery**—30 seconds to 2 minutes between sets; 48 hours between workouts

- **Progression**—During the first three weeks of your program, attempt to increase the number of reps per set as your fitness level improves—for example, start with ten reps and progress to twenty reps. After you've increased the rep count to twenty, increase the number of sets per exercise from 1 to 2 for three weeks, then add a third set to each exercise.

STAGE 2: INTERMEDIATE STAGE

This is the transitional period between the initial muscular-endurance building stage and a more demanding muscular-strength building stage.

- **Number of exercises**—Same as base-training stage
- **Intensity**—70–80 percent 1RM or 10RM
- **Duration**—8–12 reps, 2–3 sets per exercise
- **Frequency**—Same as base-training stage
- **Recovery**—Same as base-training stage
- **Progression**—As you did with the base-training stage, begin by increasing the number of reps per set as your fitness level improves; then, increase the weight to 80 percent of 1RM. Begin with 2 sets and progress to 3 sets by the end of this stage.

STAGE 3: ADVANCED STAGE

This is the muscular-strength building stage, characterized by heavy weight and low repetitions.

- **Number of exercises**—No more than 8 for all major muscle groups per workout.
- **Intensity**—80–90 percent 1RM or 1–2 levels above 10RM
- **Duration**—5–8 reps, 2–4 sets—split routine (alternate between different muscle groups each workout; for example, upper body one day, lower body the next day, then repeat) when the total number of sets reaches 20 or more

- **Frequency**—2–3 times per week for total body workouts, 4–5 per week for split routines
- **Recovery**—2–5 minutes between sets, 48–72 hours between workouts
- **Progression**—Increasing the intensity from 80 percent to 90 percent is more important than increasing the number of repetitions or the number of sets with constant resistance.

STAGE 4: MAINTENANCE STAGE

This is a combination of muscular endurance and muscular strength training with moderate to heavy weight and a moderate number of repetitions.

- **Number of exercises**—10–15 exercises per workout
- **Intensity**—70–85 percent 1RM
- **Duration**—8–12 reps, 1–3 sets
- **Frequency**—2–3 times per week
- **Recovery**—2–3 minutes between sets, 48–72 hours between workouts
- **Progression**—None

STAGE 5: RECOVERY STAGE

The recovery stage is an essential part of muscle development. During the recovery stage, your body is given a chance to recover from the stress you've placed upon it and/or any injuries. As a result, it will respond better to the next weight training cycle. If you decide to engage in exercise, keep it very light.

- **Number of exercises**—however many you feel you'd like to do
- **Intensity**—65–75 percent
- **Duration**—10–20 reps, 1–3 sets per exercise
- **Frequency**—1–3 times per week
- **Recovery**—2–4 minutes between sets
- **Progression**—None

MOVING THROUGH THE STAGES

Each stage should continue for at least four weeks and should be followed by a rest or recovery week. A fifth stage, or recovery stage, can be added after the completion of all four stages. You do not need to spend longer than three months on any one particular stage. The advanced stage should be the shortest one of all, lasting no longer than six weeks. The entire weight-training cycle—from base training to recovery stage—should take you 6–12 months to complete. Each time you start a new cycle, proceed in the same order. Do not skip any of the stages, including the recovery stage, as this would increase your chances of overtraining, burnout, and/or injury.

Base-Training Stage

This stage of your weight-training program lasts 4–8 weeks. It is characterized by training with lower resistance levels and higher repetitions. The more time you spend building the base, the stronger your foundation will be. There is no need, however, to spend longer than three months building your base.

This training program will allow you to improve your muscular endurance with a minimal amount of discomfort and soreness. This will also allow you to prepare for the more advanced strength training to come. You will start with one set per exercise, and every one or two weeks, try to raise the number of sets until you get to a maximum of 4 sets. However, for this stage, 3 sets per exercise is ideal. The total number of reps should never increase above 20. If the number of repetitions is above 20, it is time to increase the weight or resistance.

> Retest yourself following a recovery week after the completion of each stage. Use these new standards to restructure your routine.

Intermediate Stage

During the intermediate stage, which should last 4–6 weeks, the number of sets will stay steady at 2–3. At the beginning of each subsequent stage, as the percentage of resistance goes up, you should lower the number of sets performed for the first 2 or 3 weeks. Start with 2 sets per exercise and use a higher percentage of your maximum (70–80 percent 1RM) or use your present 10RM level. This means you will be able to execute a lower number of repetitions (fewer than 15 reps). An ideal level of resistance will allow you to complete a set of 8–12 reps. As you get stronger, the number of reps will go up. Once you are able to do 3 sets of 12, it is time to increase the weight.

Advanced Stage

This stage will require more energy during training as well as longer recovery time. This stage lasts 4-6 weeks. Do not attempt to train at this level of intensity for longer than that. Make sure you complete this stage prior to your competitive season (if that is your goal), or you will not be able to perform up to your potential. This kind of training should be done during the off-season or in pre-season. Never weight train the day before an important event. Consider taking at least two days off from weight training before a competition.

In general, during the advanced stage, the intensity of resistance will be 80–90 percent 1RM or 1–2 levels higher than 10RM. The number of reps is fewer than 10. The number of sets is 2–4. It is essential during this stage to split the routine among several body parts and a limited total number of exercises per workout (2–3 body parts and fewer than 8 exercises). The rest period between sets is longer than it is during the base or intermediate stages. The recovery time between sessions is 2–3 days as necessary.

> If you are a competitive athlete who competes regularly, be extra cautious when weight training. Take at least one day, preferably two days, off from weight training before a tournament. For more information, review the recovery guidelines in Chapter 2.

Maintenance Stage

It is important to include the maintenance stage in your training cycle. You may be tempted to prolong the advanced stage because you feel strong or because you feel pressured by your peers or coaches to do so. However, there is a fine line between overloading and overtraining. Overloading is a normal part of the training process, which leads to incremental increases in strength. But if you continue to increase the load for too long, you will reach a point of diminishing returns in which case you will see minimal or no improvement and possibly a decrease in performance. The maintenance stage allows you to stay strong and sharp without much risk of overtraining.

If at any time during the course of training you realize that you do not have enough time or desire to train as hard as necessary to improve, you may start your maintenance stage. If you can at least maintain your new level of muscular strength or muscular endurance, you won't have to start from the beginning when you resume your weight-training cycle. In this case, the maintenance stage can act as a temporary recovery period.

Recovery Stage

This stage is needed to allow your body to completely recover from the rigors of training and competition during the year. Take off as many days as you need during the week until you feel refreshed. Exercise no more than 3 times per week at low intensity (65–75 percent 1RM) with high repetitions (12–20 reps) and long rest periods (2–4 minutes). You do not need more than 4 weeks to recover from one full cycle of weight training.

Recovery time between sets should be at least as long as the guidelines recommend. You may take a longer break between sets if you feel unable to complete the same number of reps as with the previous set. A shorter recovery phase will result in a more intense workout, which might not be in your best interest.

CONCLUSION

Dividing your year into training stages helps you develop specific areas of muscle fitness most effectively with minimal risk of injury or overtraining. It also allows you to gauge your progress more efficiently. Recognizing when to switch from one training stage to the next will take some time, but with the proper attention, you'll learn this "fine art." Because of individual differences, it may take you longer to adapt to each stage than it may for someone else. Don't compare yourself to others. Above all, be careful not to progress too quickly, as this might set you back a lot longer than an extra week of training at a more basic stage.

CHAPTER 4

Lower-Body Exercises

The lower body is the foundation upon which the upper body rests. This means that it is as important, if not more important, to expend as much effort working on the muscles in the lower part of your body as you do on the upper part of your body. A common mistake that martial artists make is overdeveloping the upper body—especially the arms—because it is used for punching and blocking. However, it is a strong lower body that allows for more powerful upper-body techniques.

This chapter includes a full description of the lower-body exercises that an average martial artist will find most beneficial. These descriptions include the muscle group a particular exercise develops as well as its relevance to martial arts training. Your lower-body routine will consist of squats (arguably the most important multi-joint exercise there is), leg extensions, leg curls, heel raises, ankle flexion, multi-hip exercises, and hip-adductor/hip-abductor exercises. Keep in mind that it takes time to realize how a muscle feels when it is stressed. So be sure to learn the proper technique and recognize the proper sensation of the stressed muscle.

For many of the exercises described in this chapter, you'll need access to gym equipment. You can identify these exercises by the symbol ⚖. In most cases, an alternative method of working out that particular muscle group is also included.

SQUATS

Major muscle groups involved—Isolates the front of thigh (quadriceps) and the buttocks (gluteus maximus); also strengthens the lower back and the leg muscles.

Relevance to the martial arts—Performing squats translates into stronger and more stable stances, as well as improved side and back kicks.

Alternative methods of training—Leg presses (see page 31), lunges (see page 32)

Execution—The squat can be performed from a ready position (feet shoulder width apart) or from an extra-wide stance to emulate the horse stance. In either case, start with your feet apart and the bar placed firmly on your shoulders (see Figure 4.1). Make sure you have a firm grip on the barbell. Squat down until your knees achieve a ninety-degree angle (see Figure 4.2). Your upper body naturally leans forward as you squat; don't try to keep it erect.

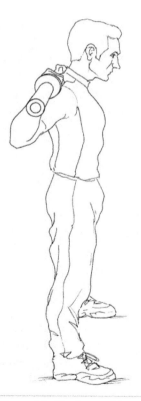

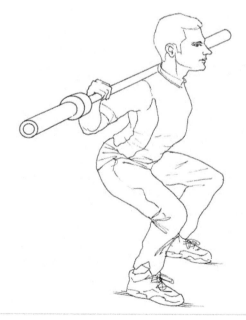

Figure 4.1. Starting position for the squat.

Figure 4.2. Finishing position for the squat.

This is the single-most important lower-body exercise. Extra care should be taken to learn the proper form. If performed incorrectly, this exercise is potentially riskier than any other exercise. Therefore, to master the technique initially, perform this exercise without any weight and keep your hands in front of your body.

Once you begin to lift weights, this exercise should not be performed without the assistance of a spotter. The spotter should not interfere unless he or she sees you struggling. If you start to struggle, your spotter should position him- or herself directly behind you. In order for the spotter to be effective and safe, he or she should squat along with you, keeping their hands positioned under the barbell, applying just enough pressure to help you lift the weight back up.

ALTERNATIVES TO SQUATS

Leg Presses

This exercise requires access to gym equipment, but it is a less-risky alternative to squats. Depending on the specific model or brand of equipment, leg presses can be performed in a seated or a supine position (see Figure 4.3). In either case, start with your knees bent at a ninety-degree angle. Push the footplate away from your body until your legs are fully extended. Do not, however, lock your knees completely at the finish; doing so provides a temporary rest period, which you do not want, and puts undue stress on your knee joints. Instead, you should be feeling constant resistance until the muscle fatigues toward the end of the set.

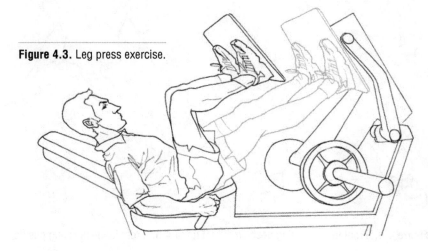

Figure 4.3. Leg press exercise.

Lunges

Lunges are also a less risky alternative to squats and don't require access to gym equipment. However, this exercise can be done in conjunction with the squat or leg press. Remember, the more exercises you perform for each body part, the more stress you place on the muscle group. In any event, squats, leg presses, and lunges are essentially working the same muscle groups so it is not necessary to perform all three during the same workout.

To execute a proper lunge, begin in a ready position with your hands at your sides (see Figure 4.4). Step out with either leg as you would for a regular front stance. Bend your knee to a right angle, then return to a ready position (see Figures 4.5 and 4.6). Once you've completed the set on one side of your body, complete the set on the other side. You can start by doing this exercise without any extra weight. As you get stronger and more experienced, you can use a set of dumbbells or a barbell.

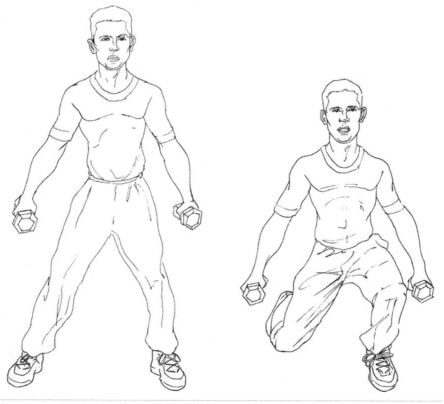

Figure 4.4. Front lunge starting position.   **Figure 4.5.** Front lunge finishing position.

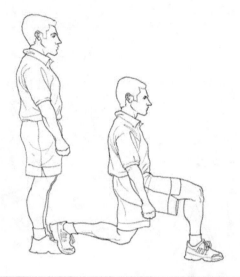

Figure 4.6. Side view of the front lunge.

⚜ LEG EXTENSIONS

Major muscle groups involved—Isolates the front of thighs (quadriceps), the muscle group that allows for the upward movement of the leg.

Relevance to the martial arts—Performing leg extensions improves the power and effectiveness of front kicks and round kicks.

Alternative methods of training—Seated extensions with ankle weights (see below).

Execution—Before beginning, make sure to adjust the seat and the back pad so that there is very little room, if any, between the back of your knee and the seat pad. The leg pad should be slightly above your foot, resting on the lower part of your shinbone (see Figure 4.7).

To perform this exercise, sit up, gripping the side edges of the seat or the handles with both hands. With your feet slightly apart, slowly raise the pad and elevate your legs until they are fully extended. Lock your knees and pause for a split second at the top. Then slowly lower your feet without allowing the plates to touch the weight stack.

> **Seated Extensions with Ankle Weights.** Sit on a firm chair with hands grasping the sides of the seat and feet flat on the floor shoulder-width apart. Raise your legs—fitted with ankle weights—until they are parallel to the floor. Pause, then lower legs back to the starting position for one rep.

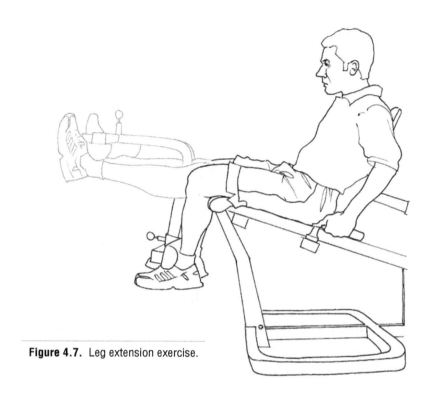

Figure 4.7. Leg extension exercise.

LEG FLEXION/LEG CURLS

Major muscle groups involved—Isolates the back of thighs (hamstrings). When trying to improve the strength in the front of the thigh, you also need to strengthen the back of the thigh to avoid the potential imbalance. Leg flexion/leg curl exercises accomplish this objective. This exercise also strengthens the buttocks (gluteus maximus) and the leg muscles below the knee, mainly the calves.

Relevance to the martial arts—This exercise improves the ability to retrieve your kicks after they have hit their target. This can help you avoid getting caught by your opponent on the way back.

Alternative methods of training—Pelvic raises (see page 35), standing leg curls with ankle weights (see page 36).

Execution—Before beginning, make sure the machine is properly adjusted

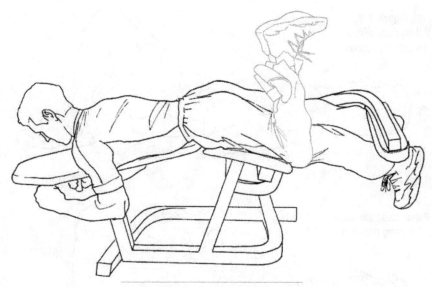

Figure 4.8. Leg curl exercise.

to your size. To perform this exercise, assume a prone position with your hands gripping the edge or the handles along the side of the bench (see Figure 4.8). Your ankles should be placed under the pad with your knees resting just below the lower end of the bench. To begin, raise your heels as far as possible toward your buttocks without lifting your buttocks to avoid strain on your lower back. Pause at the top, then lower the weight without allowing the plates to touch.

To learn the proper form, you can start by using ankle weights instead of the machine, but for this exercise to be most effective, it's best to use gym equipment.

ALTERNATIVES TO LEG FLEXION

Pelvic Raises

To perform pelvic raises, lie on your back with your knees bent, feet flat on the floor, and hands at your sides (see Figure 4.9). Elevate your pelvic region as high as you can without placing undue stress on your neck and shoulders, while tensing your back, buttock, and hamstring muscles. Hold the position for a count of two, then return to the starting position. For a complete set, perform 10–15 reps.

Figure 4.9.
Pelvic raise exercise,
starting position.

Pelvic raise exercise,
finishing position.

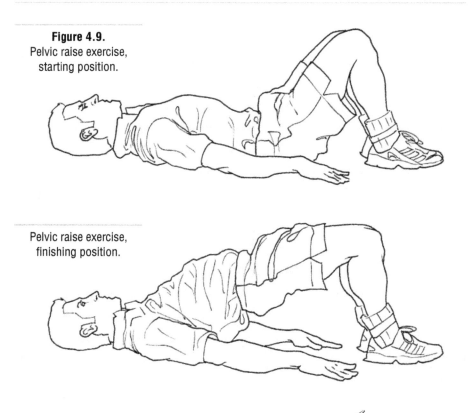

Standing Leg Curls with Ankle Weights

Place a 5–10 pound ankle weight on each ankle, and stand with your feet slightly apart. Shift all your weight to one leg, and flex the hamstring muscles of your other leg to lift up your heel until your lower leg is parallel to the floor. Hold this position for a second, and then lower your foot to the ground (see Figure 4.10). If you need help balancing during this exercise, hold on to something stable.

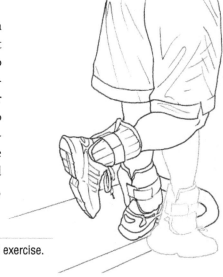

Figure 4.10. Standing leg curl exercise.

⟨⟩ STANDING HEEL RAISES

Major muscle groups involved—Isolates the calf muscle (gastrocnemius).

Relevance to the martial arts—The calf muscle is responsible for extending the foot for a better reach in front kicks and round kicks. Strengthening this muscle will improve your movement, agility, and leaping ability.

Alternative methods of training—Seated heel raises (see page 38).

Execution—Perform this exercise in a standing position (see Figure 4.11). Go up on your toes, raising your heels off the floor, and then place them back down (see Figure 4.12). You can do this exercise with both feet at the same time or, to increase the resistance, exercise one leg at a time.

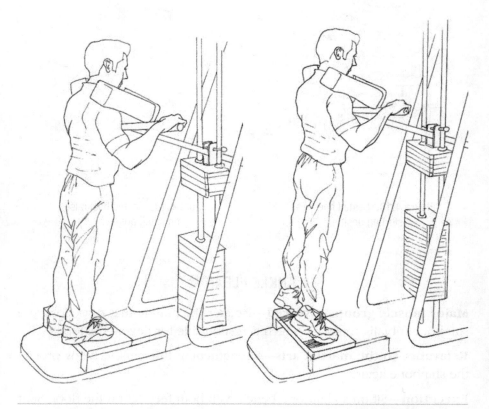

Figure 4.11. Heel raise exercise starting position.

Figure 4.12. Heel raise exercise finishing position.

ALTERNATIVE TO STANDING HEEL RAISES

🔺 *Seated Heel Raises*

From a sitting position with your knees under the pads and the ball of your feet resting on the foot platform, raise your heels up and down by contracting the calf muscles (see Figures 4.13 and 4.14).

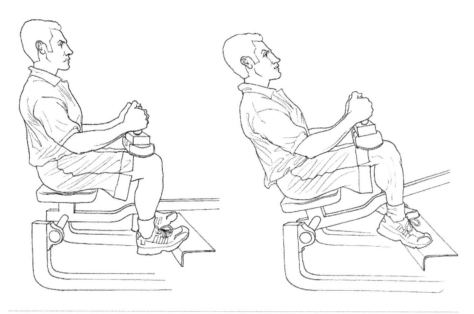

Figure 4.13. Seated heel raise starting position.

Figure 4.14. Seated heel raise finishing position.

ANKLE FLEXION

Major muscle groups involved—Isolates the muscle that runs along the shinbone (tibialis anterior), which is responsible for flexing the foot.

Relevance to the martial arts—Strengthening this muscle helps protect the shinbone against injury.

Execution—Sit on a chair or a bench with both feet flat on the floor. Start by placing a single 10-pound weight plate on top of both feet. Flex the feet at the same time, and then place them back down for a single repetition.

◢◣ MULTI-HIP EXERCISES

Major muscle groups involved— Isolates the buttocks (gluteus maximus).

Relevance to the martial arts—This exercise improves the effectiveness of back kicks and side kicks.

Alternative methods of training— Squats (see page 30), back kicks with ankle weights (see below), step-ups (see below), or back kicks on the glute master (see page 40).

Execution—Position yourself in front of the elevated lever attachment (see Figure 4.15). Place your leg on top of the lever pad with your knee flexed. Then lower your foot to the ground beside the one you are standing on. Do not try to overextend or arch your back. To work the other side, face the opposite direction.

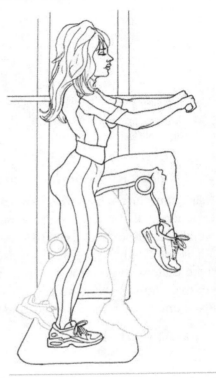

Figure 4.15. Multi-hip exercise.

ALTERNATIVES TO MULTI-HIP EXERCISES

Back Kicks with Ankle Weights

Place a 5–10 pound ankle weight on each ankle. Position yourself on all fours (see Figure 4.16). Kick your heel back on one side, hold your leg up for a count of two, and then bring your leg back to the starting position. Finish the set on one side and then perform on the other side.

Step-Ups. Stand next to a flat bench or step. Step up with one foot and then bring up your other foot so that you are standing on the bench or step with both feet. Then, step backward off of the bench with the foot you started with for one rep. Repeat the exercise using the opposite foot first. You can use dumbbells for added resistance.

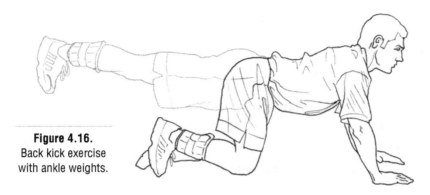

Figure 4.16.
Back kick exercise
with ankle weights.

Back Kicks on the Glute Master Machine

Using the glute master machine can be a tricky and somewhat awkward experience. If you are uncomfortable using it, simply avoid it and use ankle weights as described above. However, if you decide to use it, be sure to adjust the height of the stomach pad so that your supporting thigh forms a right angle with your torso. Position yourself atop the chest pad with both elbows and one knee atop the elbow and knee rests (see Figure 4.17). Place one foot on the footplate and push it up until the thigh is in line with

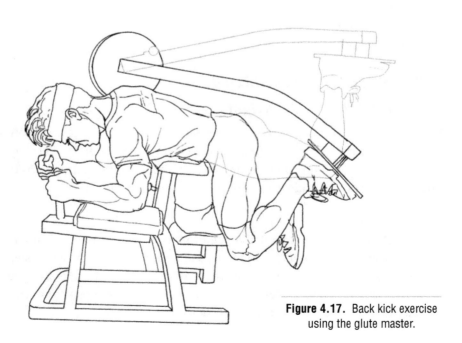

Figure 4.17. Back kick exercise
using the glute master.

the torso. Then lower your knee for one repetition. Perform the same exercise with other leg.

⁄4⁀ HIP ADDUCTION/HIP ABDUCTION

Major muscle groups involved—Isolates inner thigh muscles (adductors) and outer thigh muscles (abductors).

Relevance to the martial arts—Developing your adductor muscles helps improve the effectiveness of your sweeps, and developing your abductor muscles, which allow you to raise your legs to the side, improves your side kicks and round kicks.

Alternative methods of training—For abductor muscles, lateral leg lifts with ankle weights or bands; for adductor muscle, reverse action with ankle weights or the bands. (These exercises are not described herein.)

Execution—You can work these muscle groups either on adductor/abductor equipment or on the multi-hip machine. To strengthen your inner thigh on the adductor/abductor machine, begin with your knees apart and then bring them together for a single repetition (see Figures 4.18 and 4.19). To

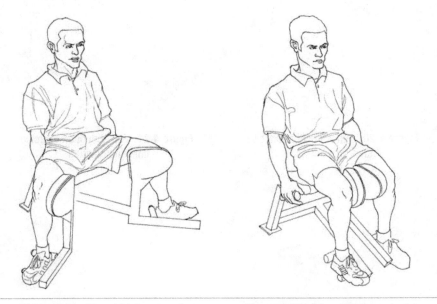

Figure 4.18. Hip adduction exercise starting position.

Figure 4.19. Hip adduction exercise finishing position.

strengthen the outer thigh muscle, perform the opposite action of the adductor muscle. Start with your feet together and spread your legs apart and back together to complete a repetition (see Figures 4.20 and 4.21). You do not need to spread your legs too far apart. Remember, you are not stretching the muscles; you're building them. Spreading your legs too far apart could cause injury.

This muscle is relatively weak as well, so you do not have to use too much weight. Start with the lowest resistance possible and increase the resistance when you are able to complete at least 10 repetitions successfully.

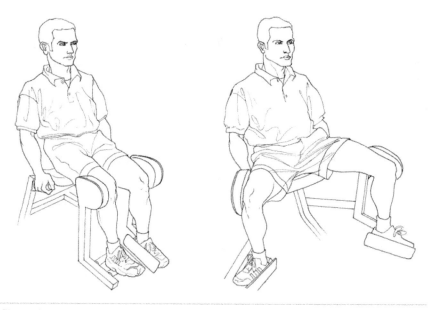

Figure 4.20. Hip abduction exercise starting position.

Figure 4.21. Hip abduction exercise finishing position.

Table 4.1 lists the most popular lower-body exercises.

TABLE 4.1. LOWER-BODY EXERCISES		
Body Part	**Exercises**	
Quadriceps (front of thigh)	• Leg presses	• Lunges
	• Squats	• Leg extensions
Hamstrings (back of thigh)	• Leg flexion/leg curls	• Lunges
	• Back extensions	• Squats
Calves (back of the leg below the knee)	• Heel raises/foot extension	
Tibialis anterior (front of the leg below the knee)	• Ankle flexion	
Gluteus maximus (buttocks)	• Multi-hip exercises	• Lunges
	• Squats/leg presses	
Hip flexors	• Sit-ups	

CONCLUSION

It's very important to familiarize yourself with all of these exercises during the first month of your training program. Be sure to incorporate them into your weekly routine. You'll find that you may like some and dislike others. But don't give up on an exercise simply because you don't like it. Chances are, it's working the muscles where you need it most.

Make sure to spend an equal amount of time developing opposing muscle groups to avoid overdeveloping one area. A significant discrepancy between opposing muscle groups can lead to pesky injuries that will haunt you for the rest of your martial arts career. As it is in just about everything in life, balance is very important in the martial arts.

Keep in mind that lower-body work takes lots of energy, so be sure to take extra time to recover between your workouts.

CHAPTER 5

Upper-Body Exercises

Martial arts training, especially karate training, can contribute a great deal to the overall upper-body development. After all, the average student of the martial arts performs dozens of punching and blocking techniques, not to mention dozens of push-ups and sit-ups during every training session. This appears to be enough to cover all bases, but when we analyze the situation a little closer, we find that there are lots of missing parts. For starters, most martial arts techniques recruit the muscles in the front of the upper body, primarily the pectoral region (the chest), the deltoid muscles (the front of the shoulder), and the triceps (the back of the upper arm), as well as the obliques (abdominal region or the stomach muscles). As a result, this area of the body is well developed.

However, the problem is that the back muscles tend to be underdeveloped compared with the front of the body. This creates an imbalance between the two regions, with the lower back being more susceptible to injury. The lower lumbar region on the back, which is one of the most delicate areas in our bodies, is so vulnerable because martial arts training does nothing to strengthen it. Worse yet, doing many of the moves that a karate student is required to do can actually damage the lower back, creating injuries that can take weeks and sometimes months to heal. Therefore, martial artists cannot do enough for their back muscles. It is absolutely imperative that we take time to strengthen the entire back region to correct the imbalance. Three of the best exercises that achieve this objective are pull-ups or pull-downs, seated rows, and back extensions.

Another drawback with martial arts training is the lack of muscle-strength building. The only kind of resistance training that is done is calisthenics, more specifically push-ups. The downside of this type of training is that it improves one's muscular endurance system without improving one's muscular strength. If you want to consider yourself a complete martial artist, it is imperative to develop muscular strength as well as muscular endurance. For this purpose, the chest press is one of the best exercises to perform. Performed on a flat bench, the chest press is very effective in improving the strength of your chest, shoulder, and triceps muscles (the very same muscle areas stressed when performing regular push-ups). With push-ups, however, you are limited by your own body weight. Furthermore, most students can perform in excess of 20 repetitions at one time. This makes it ineffective for improving one's muscular strength because the resistance level is not high enough to stress the muscular strength system. With chest presses, you can adjust the weight to any desirable resistance level. Selecting heavy resistance (80–90 percent 1RM) and performing fewer repetitions (5–10 reps) will allow you to work primarily on your muscular strength.

Another important upper-body exercise that works a relatively large muscle area is the overhead or shoulder press. Other exercises include lateral raises, biceps curls, and triceps push-downs. These work smaller muscle groups in the body such as the deltoids, the biceps, and the triceps. In any event, this chapter includes a full description of the upper-body exercises that an average martial artist will find most beneficial. These descriptions include the specific muscle group a particular exercise develops as well as its relevance to martial arts training.

> For many of the exercises described in this chapter, you'll need access to gym equipment. You can identify these exercises by the symbol ⚍. In most cases, an alternative method of working that particular muscle group is also included.

Keep in mind that it takes time to realize how a muscle feels when it is stressed. So be sure learn the proper technique and recognize the proper sensation of the stressed muscle.

MULTIJOINT OR LARGE MUSCLE GROUPS

 PULL-DOWNS

Major muscle groups involved—Isolates the upper and middle back (latissimus dorsi and the rhomboids), the back of the shoulders (posterior deltoid), and the front of the arm (biceps).

Relevance to the martial arts—Injury prevention from improper posture due to uneven muscle development.

Alternative methods of training—Pull-ups (see Figures 5.4 and 5.5) are an alternative to this exercise if you are strong enough to execute five or more without assistance.

Execution—There are several ways to perform pull-downs. Here are two of them: wide-grip or reverse-grip pull-downs. Both ways are useful and strengthen slightly different muscle groups in the upper back.

To do the wide-grip pull-downs, use the overhand grip with your palms facing away from you and your hands wider than shoulder width or approximately 20 to 30 inches apart (see Figures 5.1 and 5.2). To do the

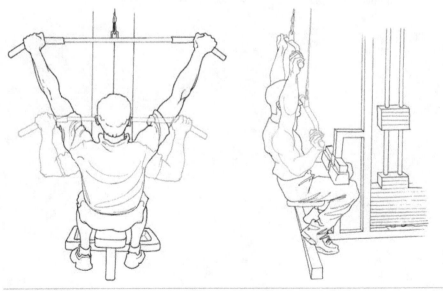

Figure 5.1. Wide-grip pull-down exercise (posterior view).   **Figure 5.2.** Wide-grip pull-down exercise (side view).

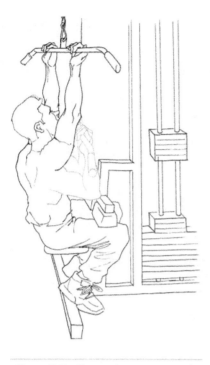

Figure 5.3. Close-grip or reverse-grip pull-down exercise.

reverse grip pull-downs, use an underhand grip with your hands about 10–20 inches apart (see Figure 5.3). Using either grip, pull the bar down until it is just underneath your chin and then slowly return the bar to the starting position. Try not to pause at the top or bottom of the pull-downs. Do not lower the bar below your shoulders. If you do, you will be engaging other weaker muscles and not overloading the targeted muscles. Take special care to minimize your upper-body movement. Do not rock back and forth with each repetition.

If you do both wide grip and reverse grip during your routine, you won't have to do any other exercise for your upper back. Start with one set of wide-grip pull-downs, rest for 2–3 minutes, and then complete another set of pull-downs using the reverse grip.

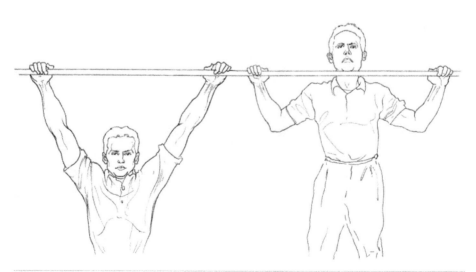

Figure 5.4. Wide-grip pull-up exercise starting position.

Figure 5.5. Wide-grip pull-up exercise finishing position.

↳⟨↿∧↾⟨ SEATED ROWS

Major muscle groups involved—Isolates the upper middle back (rhomboids), the back of the shoulder (posterior deltoid), and the top of arm (biceps). This exercise also engages the erector muscles that support your spine.

Relevance to the martial arts—Corrects muscle imbalance.

Alternative methods of training—Reverse grip pull-down (see page 48), bent-over dumbbell rows (see page 50).

Execution—Perform this exercise in a seated position with your legs almost completely extended (see Figure 5.6). Maintain erect upper-body posture, with your arms fully extended, your shoulders back, and your chest out. Use your back and biceps muscles to pull the weight toward you while keeping the rest of your body as still as possible. Stick your chest out as you pull your hands toward you. When your elbows are at a right angle, hold for a moment and then slowly return the weight back to the starting point. Pay strict attention to your form, making sure your shoulders do not rise and you do not rock your torso back and forth.

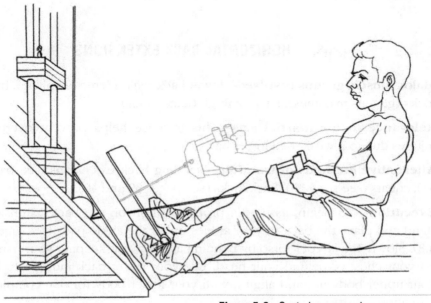

Figure 5.6. Seated row exercise.

ALTERNATIVE TO SEATED ROWS

Bent-Over Dumbbell Rows

To perform bent-over dumbbell rows, begin by posi-
tioning the knee and hand
on the supporting side
of your body on a flat
bench (see Figure 5.7).
Your torso should be
parallel to the floor.
The arm performing
the exercise should
be fully extended,
firmly gripping the
dumbbell. Pull the
dumbbell up to-

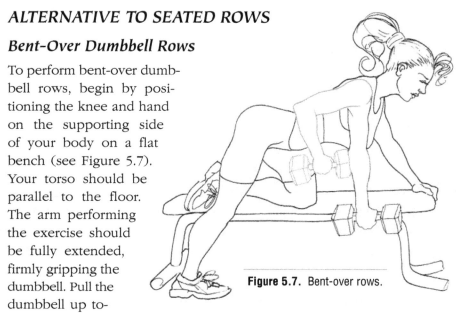

Figure 5.7. Bent-over rows.

ward your side until your upper arm is parallel to the floor and your elbow
achieves a ninety-degree angle, then slowly lower the dumbbell to the
starting position for one rep. Keep your body as still as possible while performing this exercise. Perform on the other side.

⟨4⟩ HORIZONTAL BACK EXTENSIONS

Major muscle groups involved—lower back region (erector spinae), buttocks (gluteus maximus), back of thigh (hamstrings).

Relevance to the martial arts—This exercise helps prevent overuse
injuries due to a weakened lower back.

Alternative methods of training—Standing back extensions (see page
51), squats (see page 30), back kicks (see pages 39 and 40).

Execution—To begin, assume a prone position on the back extension
stand and place the back of your ankles under the ankle pads (see Figure
5.8). Slowly lower your torso by bending at the waist, keeping your hands
on your chest or behind your head. Use your lower back muscles to lift
your upper body up, and align it with your lower body for one complete
repetition.

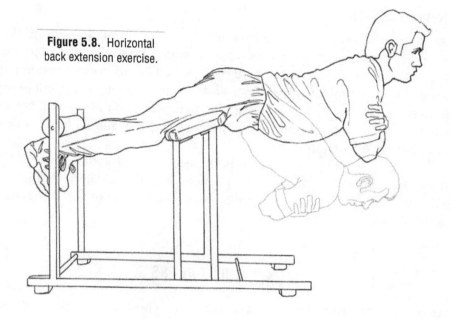

Figure 5.8. Horizontal back extension exercise.

ALTERNATIVES TO HORIZONTAL BACK EXTENSIONS

Standing Back Extensions

If you don't have access to a stand, you can still do back extensions. Start in a ready position with your knees slightly bent and your arms crossed over your chest (see Figure 5.9). Slowly bend at the waist, keeping your upper back perfectly flat and without disturbing the natural arch in your lower back. Your finishing point is when you feel you can no longer maintain a flat back. Return to a ready position to complete the repetition.

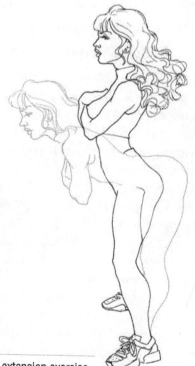

Figure 5.9. Standing back extension exercise.

Reverse Sit-Up

Another good exercise for the back is the reverse sit-up. To perform this exercise, begin by lying on your stomach with a firm pillow or large ball just below your waist. Arms should be stretched out in front of you in the superman position. Lift your upper body off the floor by contracting the muscles in your back, then return to the starting position. Be careful not to overextend by arching your back too much. The arch should be no more than the natural arch in your back.

The reverse sit-up can also be performed on the Nautilus Rotary Ab/Back Machine or a similar type of equipment with the addition of weights. Remember not to use too much weight in the beginning of your program, as this is a delicate body part.

CHEST PRESS

Major muscle groups involved—Isolates the chest muscle (pectoral region), the front of shoulder (anterior), and the back of upper arm (triceps).

Relevance to the martial arts—Improves punching and blocking power.

Alternative methods of training—Chest flyes (see page 53).

Execution—This exercise can be performed either with free weights or on a peck-deck/chest-flye machine. If you are using free weights, you must have a spotter as this exercise can be potentially dangerous. The spotter is responsible for helping you lift the weight up initially and for assisting you with the last repetition if you are not able to push the weight up on your own. The spotter should be positioned behind you with his or her feet shoulder-width apart and knees slightly bent. To assist with the last repetition, the spotter should place both hands under the bar, helping you push the weight up. When using dumbbells, the spotter should be kneeling down for better leverage and assist you by pushing up on your elbows as you attempt to execute the last repetition. The same rule applies to the chest flye exercise.

To perform the chest press, start by lying on your back with your arms fully extended and the weight evenly distributed on both sides (see Figure 5.10 on page 53). This is very important for balance especially with free weights. If you are using a barbell, both of your hands should be equi-

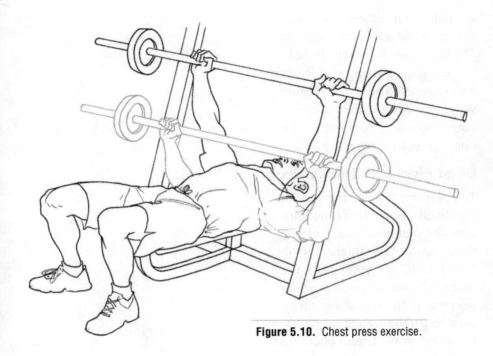

Figure 5.10. Chest press exercise.

distant from the center of the barbell. Once you have a firm grip of the bar or the dumbbells, gently lower the weight to your chest. To avoid injury, do not bounce the bar off your chest and do not arch your back excessively. Then, extend your arms as you push the weight up in one fluid motion. If you are using the barbell, allow your spotter to help you set the bar back on the rack. With dumbbells, lower them to your chest and sit up before putting them down. Do not simply release your grip and drop them on the floor. You can either hurt yourself or someone else who is standing close to you. Remember, safety first.

ALTERNATIVES TO CHEST PRESS

Chest Flyes on Chest-Flye Machine

The chest flye exercise is an isolation exercise because it isolates the chest muscle (pectoralis major) without engaging the shoulders or the triceps. To use the chest flye machine correctly, be sure to adjust the height of the seat so that your elbows are just below shoulder level. Start by placing your forearms behind the arm pads, leaving your chest area exposed. Then, slowly bring your arms toward the middle of your body and back again for one rep (see Figure 5.11).

Chest Flyes with Dumbbells

To perform chest flyes with dumbbells, begin by firmly gripping the dumbbells and holding them against your thighs. Lie on a flat bench, and gently place the dumbbells on your chest while keeping a tight grip on them. Now, push the weight up directly above you. Then, open up your chest as you gently lower both arms to the side, keeping your elbow slightly bent and your hands with your palms turned upward. Lower the weight until your upper arm is parallel to the

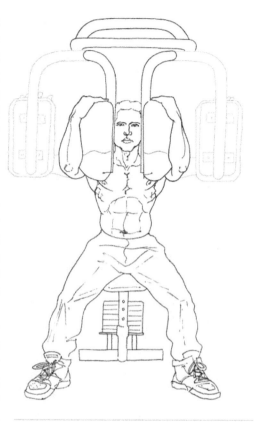

Figure 5.11. Chest flye exercise.

floor. Then slowly bring the weight back up. When the set is completed, bring both hands in toward your chest, sit up, and then place the dumbbells on the floor.

OVERHEAD PRESS

Major muscle groups involved—Isolates the shoulder muscles (deltoids) and the back of upper arm (triceps).

Relevance to the martial arts—The overhead press improves your head-blocking techniques.

Alternative methods of training—front raises, dumbbell shrugs, incline bench press (see page 55).

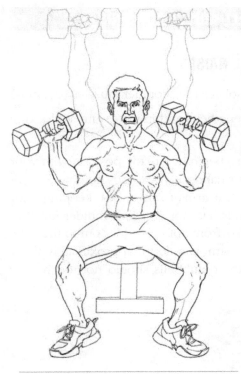

Execution—For this exercise, you can use either a standard barbell or a set of dumbbells. Start either in a seated or a standing position with your hands up and your elbows at a right angle (see Figure 5.12). Raise your hands above your head, extending your arms upward without completely locking your elbows, then slowly lower the weights to the original starting position to complete one repetition.

● ● ● ● ● ● ● ● ● ● ● ●
When you are working
with weights, remember
to keep constant pressure
on the muscle throughout
the repetition.
● ● ● ● ● ● ● ● ● ● ● ● ● ● ● ● ● ● ●

Figure 5.12. Seated overhead press exercise.

Front Raises, Dumbbell Shrugs, and Incline Bench Press

To perform **front raises**, stand with your feet shoulder-width apart and knees bent slightly. Allow your arms to hang in front of your body with each hand holding a dumbbell. Using your shoulders, lift your arms out and away from your body, until your hands reach shoulder level. Lower your arms to the starting position for one rep.

To perform **dumbbell shrugs**, stand with feel shoulder-width apart with dumbbells at your sides. Elevate, or shrug, your shoulders as high as possible. Then lower for one rep.

To perform **incline bench press**, sit on an incline bench with the dumbbells resting on your lower thighs. Bring the dumbbells to your shoulders and lean back. Press the dumbbells up with your elbows until your arms are extended. Lower weight to the sides of your upper chest for one rep.

SINGLE-JOINT/SMALL MUSCLE GROUPS

LATERAL RAISES

Major muscle groups involved—Isolates the shoulder muscles (deltoids)

Relevance to the martial arts—Strengthens and improves most blocking and striking techniques.

Execution—To perform lateral raises, begin in a ready position with your knees and arms slightly bent and your hands at your sides holding a set of dumbbells (see Figure 5.13). Raise your arms to the sides, keeping your elbows slightly higher than your hands. Do not go past shoulder level. In other words, if you were to draw a line from your shoulder out to the side, the angle between that line and your arm should be approximately thirty degrees. As you lower the weight, the dumbbells should not touch your thighs.

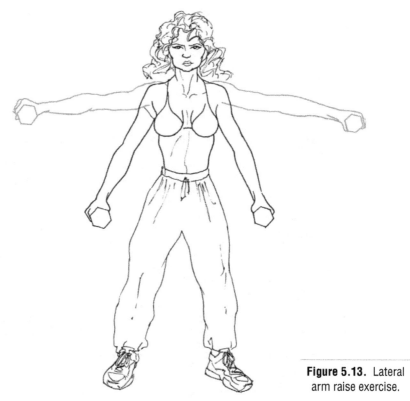

Figure 5.13. Lateral arm raise exercise.

How Much Weight to Use for Smaller Regions

You do not need to use a lot of weight to strengthen the smaller regions of your body. It is sufficient to start with light weights: 2–5 lbs for women and 3–8 lbs for men in the case of lateral raises, and 5–12 lbs for women and 8–15 lbs for men in the case of biceps and triceps exercises. Do not be intimidated by people who use much heavier weight. Chances are they are overestimating their strength level for those specific exercises and leaving themselves more susceptible to injury. However, if you perform these exercises slowly, as recommended, you will be able to strengthen those muscles with much less risk. It is important to select the right amount of resistance, use the full range of motion when lifting weights, and resist the temptation of breaking form for the sake of completing another repetition or lifting higher weight.

BICEPS CURLS

Major muscle groups involved—Isolates the upper front of arm (biceps).

Relevance to the martial arts—This is the muscle that allows you to flex your arm. Strengthening it increases your ability to retrieve your fist after a back-fist strike. It also helps to correct the imbalance in the upper arm from overdeveloped triceps muscles.

Execution—To perform this exercise, you can either use a barbell in a standing position or a set of dumbbells in a seated or a standing position. If you choose to stand, start in a ready position with your knees slightly bent, your chest out, your shoulders back, and your arms at your sides with your palms facing out (see Figure 5.14). Flex your arm as you raise the bar or the dumbbells up toward your chest, keeping constant pressure on the muscle. Pause at the top of the contraction. As you lower the weight, make sure your

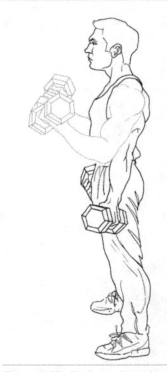

Figure 5.14. Biceps curl exercise.

arms are almost totally extended, with only a slight bend in your elbow. If you choose to sit for this exercise, the mechanics are the same. Just be sure to sit upright with your shoulders back, your chest out, and your feet together.

For Weight-Bearing Exercises Performed in a Standing Position

When you complete a set with free weights, bend at your knees to lower the weights to the ground rather than bending at your waist, which can contribute to a lower back problem.

 TRICEPS PUSH-DOWNS

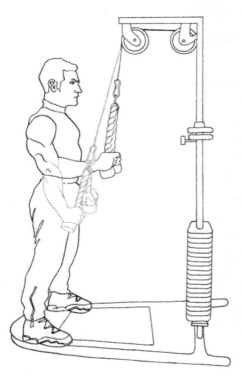

Figure 5.15. Triceps push-down exercise.

Major muscle groups involved— Isolates and strengthens the back of the upper arm (triceps).

Relevance to the martial arts— This exercise helps improve the effectiveness of most striking and blocking techniques.

Alternative methods of training— Across-the-chest triceps extensions (see page 59), dumbbell triceps extensions (see page 59).

Execution—Face the pulley machine with your feet shoulder-width apart, knees bent, shoulders back, chest out, and elbows touching the sides of your body (see Figure 5.15). You can either use the short bar or the ropes to do this exercise. Grab the bar/rope with your hands about 6–10 inches apart. Then, extend your arms and lock your elbows at the top of the contraction. Hold for a split second, and then slowly allow your forearm to rise until it is parallel to the ground and your elbow is at a right angle.

ALTERNATIVES TO TRICEPS PUSH-DOWNS ON PULLEY MACHINE

Across-the-Chest Triceps Extensions

Face the pulley machine with your feet shoulder width apart, knees bent, shoulders back, chest out, and elbows touching the sides of your body. Grab the handle with one of your hands turned sideways and bend your elbow. Your elbow should now be at your side touching your body and your fist on top of your chest (see Figure 5.16). Extend your arm to the side and lock your elbow for a split second, then slowly bring it back to the starting point for one rep.

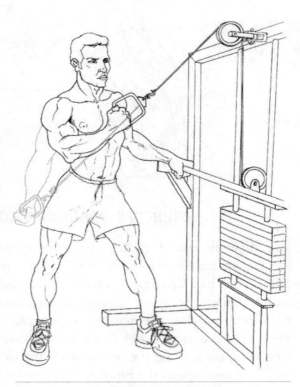

Figure 5.16. Across the chest triceps extension exercise.

Dumbbell Triceps Extension

To perform dumbbell triceps extension, begin by positioning the knee and hand on the supporting side of your body on a flat bench. Your torso should be parallel to the floor. The arm performing the exercise should be bent at a ninety-degree angle at the elbow joint, firmly gripping the dumbbell (see Figure 5.17). Fully extend your arm behind you by contracting your triceps, slowly returning to the starting position for one rep.

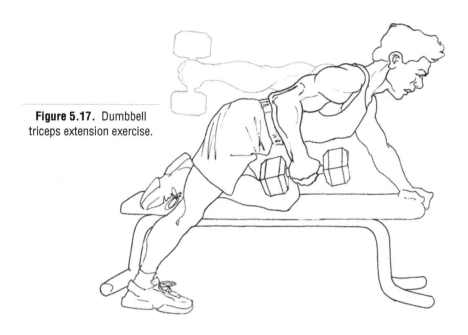

Figure 5.17. Dumbbell triceps extension exercise.

CRUNCHES (ABDOMINAL EXERCISES)

Training in the martial arts helps you to develop the strong abdominal muscles that are necessary to absorb the kicks and punches of your opponents. This doesn't mean you can't improve on the technique used to work these muscles. In practicing our kicking techniques, we tend to overdevelop our hip flexor muscles, the muscles responsible for allowing us to lift our knees. Overdeveloped hip flexor muscles are *tight* hip flexor muscles. Moreover, performing conventional sit-ups to strengthen the abdominal area tends to tighten the hip flexor muscles even more. Tight hip flexor muscles can offset your posture and cause lower back and knee injuries. What's the solution? You must perform abdominal exercises without using your hip flexor muscles and stretch the hip flexor muscles to take the pressure off the lower back and improve posture. (An excellent way to stretch your hip flexor muscles is to perform pelvic raises. This exercise is described on page 35.)

To perform crunches, choose a soft but firm surface to avoid chafing your skin. Lie flat on your back with your feet up and knees bent over your stomach (see Figure 5.18). Clasp your hands behind your head as you raise your shoulders and head off the floor while contracting your abdominal

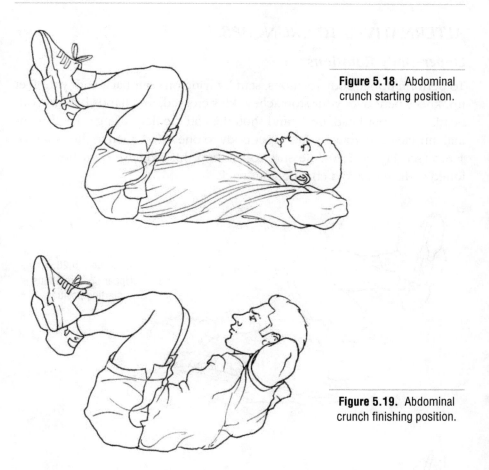

Figure 5.18. Abdominal crunch starting position.

Figure 5.19. Abdominal crunch finishing position.

muscles (see Figure 5.19). Be careful not to put any pressure on your neck by *pulling* your head forward.

If you are having difficulty performing at least ten repetitions with your hands behind your head, place your hands on your chest to make this exercise a bit easier. Perform 2–3 sets of 10–30 reps depending on your level of fitness.

Crunches are designed to strengthen your oblique muscles as well as your middle abdominal region. You only need one exercise to work your abdominal area because it's virtually impossible to isolate your upper abdominal region from your lower abdominal region. This muscle contracts as one. There is, however, a variety of abdominal exercises you can perform to change things up a bit, including upper-body rotations (see below), and bicycle kicks (see page 63).

ALTERNATIVES TO CRUNCHES

Upper-Body Rotations

To perform upper-body rotations, start by lying on your back with your feet up, knees bent over your stomach, ankles crossed, and hands behind your head. Raise your head, neck, and shoulders off the floor using your abdominal muscles, and rotate your upper body to one sided, then to the other for 1 rep (see Figure 5.20). Be sure to perform this exercise on a firm cushioned surface to avoid chafing your back.

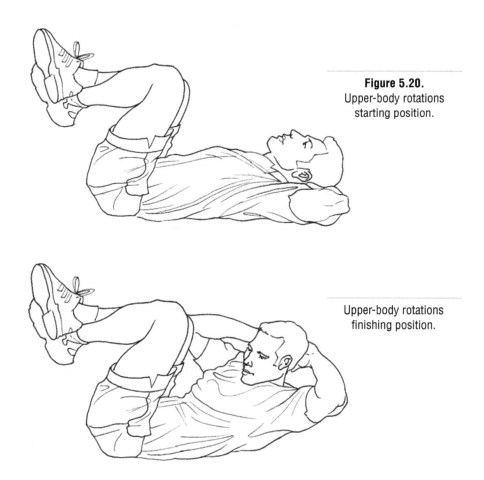

Figure 5.20.
Upper-body rotations
starting position.

Upper-body rotations
finishing position.

Bicycle Kicks

To perform bicycle kicks, start by lying on your back with your knees bent over your stomach, and hands behind your head. As you rotate your right side, reach for your left knee with your right elbow, while extending your right leg (see Figure 5.21). This is followed by the rotation of your left elbow to your right knee while extending your left leg out. Be sure to perform this exercise on a firm cushioned surface to avoid chafing your back.

Figure 5.21.
Bicycle kicks.

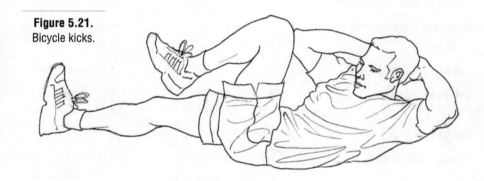

Table 5.1 presents a list of the most popular upper-body exercises.

TABLE 5.1. UPPER-BODY EXERCISES		
Body Part	**Exercises**	
Latissimus dorsi (upper back)	• Pull-downs/pull-ups	
Rhomboids (upper middle back)	• Seated rows • Bent-over rows	• Chin-ups
Erector spinae (lower back)	• Back extensions	• Reverse sit-ups
Pectoralis major (chest)	• Push-ups • Chest press	• Chest flyes • Incline press
Trapezius (shoulder)	• Shrugs	• Overhead press
Deltoids (shoulder)	• Forward/lateral/ bent-over raises	• Overhead press
Biceps (upper arm)	• Barbell/dumbbell curls	
Triceps (back of arm)	• Pulley pushdowns • Triceps extensions	• Overhead press with dumbbells or pulleys
Obliques (abdominals)	• Crunches with feet down on the floor or knees up	• Sit-ups

CONCLUSION

Most martial artists, men in particular, have a tendency to overdevelop their upper bodies, especially the chest area. Although it is very attractive to have a nicely developed pectoralis region, it is overkill to perform pushups and then on top of that, perform too many sets of weight training exercises to build even bigger chest muscles. In this chapter, we covered the areas of the upper body that often get overlooked in martial arts training—if for no other reason than a lack of proper equipment. The key is to establish a well-balanced exercise routine that covers the entire body. Even though there is a greater variety of upper-body exercises than lower-body exercises, resist the temptation to spend too much time training your upper body in general and your chest region in particular.

CHAPTER 6

Sound Sports Nutrition for the Martial Artist

Proper nutrition is an essential part of any sport or exercise program. Food is the fuel that runs the body's metabolic engine. As you can well imagine, all the preparation in the world won't help you unless you follow a sensible diet. A typical martial artist can expend more than 1,000 calories during an intense workout. Eating the right food at the right time can improve your gains in strength and endurance, while an inappropriate diet can slow your progress and leave you feeling sluggish and weak. This chapter presents you with the information you need to plan a well-balanced diet that can keep you performing at your best. In general, always listen to your body. Eat when you feel hungry, and stop before you feel full.

CARBS, FATS, AND PROTEINS

All of the food a person eats contains some combination of the three major macronutrients—carbohydrates, fats, and proteins. If consumed in the right amounts and proportions, these macronutrients supply you with all the necessary energy your body needs, and provide all of the necessary micro-nutrients, such as vitamins and minerals, to help your body function most efficiently.

Some foods have a larger proportion of one macronutrient over the other two. For example, almost all fruits, vegetables, and grains are considered carbohydrate-rich foods and contain little fat or protein. On the other hand, meat, dairy products, nuts, and seeds are made up of mostly protein and fat.

The proportions that are recommended for the average person are 50 to 60 percent carbohydrates, 10 to 20 percent proteins, and 20 to 30 percent fats. If you are a competitive athlete, your need for carbohydrates is higher. You might need 60 to 70 percent carbohydrates to keep your energy levels up.

To determine how many calories you need to consume daily to maintain your weight, multiply your weight in pounds by fifteen (if you are a man) and by thirteen (if you are a woman). That is approximately how many calories you'll need to keep up with the demands of your body without exercise. During times of intense training and competition, your caloric demand could be 300–800 calories more.

The Role of Carbohydrates in the Body

Carbohydrates—which have gotten some negative press lately due to the popularity of low-carb diets—are the body's preferred source of energy. Because it is the easiest of the macronutrients for the body to break down, carbohydrates are metabolized to produce energy before fats and proteins. Although carbohydrates are the body's most valued source of fuel, they are the least abundant of the three macronutrients in the body.

The main function of carbohydrates in the body is to provide the energy necessary to carry out physical demands, such as intense exercise and competition, and to enable the body to use fat for energy when physical intensity falls below a certain level. It is also the only fuel source for the brain and the nervous system.

Carbohydrate-Rich Foods
In addition to the general categories of carbohydrate-rich foods mentioned earlier, some of the more specific sources of carbohydrates include peas, beans, potatoes (sweet and regular), pasta, yams, rice, oats, and bran.

Because we rely so heavily on carbohydrate and because we store a relatively small amount of it in the body, we tend to run out of it much faster than the other two macronutrients. For that reason, we need to consume relatively large quantities of this nutrient on a daily basis. One gram of carbohydrates equals 4 calories of energy. To supply your body with enough energy, you need to eat roughly 400–500 grams, or in excess of 1 pound, of carbohydrate-rich foods each day.

Carbohydrates are made up of simple sugar molecules and water, but not all carbohydrates are the same. Simple carbohydrates such as table sugar and honey are made up of one or two sugar molecules. Complex carbohydrates such as beans and buckwheat are made up of several sugar molecules as well as fiber, which is necessary for maintaining proper digestion, preventing overeating, and staving off food-related illnesses such as diabetes, obesity, and heart disease.

The carbohydrates we consume daily are used either immediately for energy or to replenish our fuel tank for later use. If it is a simple form of carbohydrate it is easily and quickly digested by the body and used immediately for energy. A complex carbohydrate has to be broken down to simple form before it can be used. Therefore, complex carbohydrates are digested slowly and can provide consistent long-lasting energy throughout the day.

All sugar—whether it comes from simple or complex sources—is converted to glycogen, a complex form of sugar, if it is not used immediately for energy. We store glycogen in our muscle (approximately 325 grams), in our liver (approximately 100 grams), and in our blood in the form of glucose (approximately 20 grams). The average person's maximum capacity for glycogen storage is roughly 500 grams or 2,000 calories. This translates to a maximum of two hours of moderate-to-high intensity work.

With training, a competitive athlete can expand his capacity for glycogen storage by as much as 100 percent. This can be accomplished by high volume and/or high-intensity endurance training or by high volume low-intensity muscle endurance training. The ability to increase your capacity for glycogen storage allows you to increase your exercise capacity. This allows you to increase the duration and intensity of your workout so that you progress and get better and stronger.

The Role of Protein in the Body

The consumption of protein is necessary to build and repair muscle tissue, to regulate the acid/base quality of body fluids, for the production of enzymes, for blood clotting, for oxygen transport, and for making up your DNA. When glycogen levels are very low in extreme cases, the body can use protein for energy. This is the least desirable way to generate energy because your muscles are being broken down. If your body uses protein for energy, your body's ability to grow and increase in strength is negated.

You need to consume roughly 1–1.5 grams of protein per kilogram (2.2

pounds) of body weight per day. For a man who weighs 75 kg (165 lbs), the consumption of protein must equal 75–110 grams, or 2.5–4 ounces, of protein per day.

The best sources of protein include eggs (5 grams per ounce), lean meats (7–8 grams per ounce), fish (5–7 grams per ounce), red kidney beans (7 grams per ounce), and soybeans (10 grams per ounce).

The Role of Fat in the Body

The most abundant source of energy in the body is in the form of fat. One gram of fat can generate 9 calories of energy. That's twice as much as carbohydrates or protein. Because of this, it's ideal to rely on fat for energy whenever possible. Unfortunately for the practitioner of the martial arts, generating energy from fat is not likely. The higher the intensity of work, the more reliant the body becomes on carbohydrates and, later, on proteins. During recovery periods and at rest, the body tries to spare the most precious macronutrients and will switch to burning fat instead.

With so much fat available in the body, why is consuming dietary fat so important? Well, besides its role in providing the body with energy, fat also serves to maintain the integrity of cell walls, helps regulate certain body functions, transports and stores fat-soluble vitamins, adds flavor and texture to foods, and helps delay hunger pangs due to delayed stomach emptying. Moreover, dietary fats are the only source of the essential fats that the body does not produce on its own.

Note: if you are a competitive athlete, it might be necessary to increase your consumption of fat in the diet if you find it difficult to keep up with the caloric demands of your training program with low-fat foods.

TIMING IS EVERYTHING

Because you are an athlete in training, your dietary objectives are somewhat different from the average person's. Your challenge is not just to eat a well-balanced diet, but also to consume the right combination of food at the right time. There's a right time to consume simple carbohydrates, a right time to consume complex carbohydrates, a right time to eat more fat, and a right time to eat more protein.

For starters, most of your diet should consist of complex carbohydrates (grains, pasta, rice, potatoes, beans, breads, and so on), fruits, vegetables, and lean meats and eggs, as reflected in the sample menus on pages 71–74. The consumption of carbohydrates is especially important before, during, and after training and competition because the body's demand for sugars is much higher during bouts of physical and mental stress.

Before an intense exercise session—especially in the extreme heat— you should consume 50–100 grams of simple carbohydrates, preferably in the form of an energy drink or an energy bar. Then, every 15–30 minutes, consume 25–50 grams of simple carbohydrates, being sure to hydrate yourself. (An energy drink will provide the carbohydrates and liquid your body needs.) Your caloric needs will most likely increase due to the high level of energy expended.

Since the capacity to restore depleted glycogen supplies as well as the capacity for building muscles is much higher right after exercise than at any other time during the day, for an hour immediately following the end of the workout or competition, continue to consume 40–50 g (or 150–200 calories) of carbohydrates, but now add 20–25 grams (80–100 calories) of protein. This is not over and above your caloric requirements calculated earlier.

The consumption of fats should be limited just before, during, and right after exercise.

After about an hour of post competition or exercise, resume eating complex carbohydrates to delay gastric emptying and to slow down the use of sugars for energy. At this point, you can add more fat and protein to the meal as the body switches to fats as the primary source of energy and focuses on muscle synthesis due to higher intake of proteins.

AVOIDING GLYCOGEN DEPLETION

If we do not consume at least 1,000 calories of carbohydrate-rich food daily (approximately 50 percent of total dietary food intake), we are at risk for glycogen depletion. This is a state of physical and mental fatigue that is experienced when glycogen stores are very low—when your carbohydrate intake falls well below your body's demand for it. If you increase your exercise volume and/or intensity without a sufficient increase in your food and carbohydrate intake, you are putting yourself at risk for glycogen depletion. The only way your body can replenish its glycogen stores is through an ample supply of carbohydrates. If this does not occur for several days, your body will start using protein for energy and will conserve its limited glycogen stores. If your body is depleted of its glycogen supply for more than several days, you are at risk of developing chronic fatigue syndrome.

Under normal circumstance, when your body's glycogen supplies are significantly depleted, it takes two days of carbohydrate loading (the intake of carbohydrates above your usual percentage) and/or a decrease in exercise intensity to get your supplies back to normal. However, when you reach the point of chronic fatigue, it can take several weeks and sometimes months to get back to full reserves.

To prevent glycogen depletion, be sure to consume enough total calories every day, making sure that at least 40 percent of your total food intake is in the form of complex carbohydrates and another 10–20 percent is in the form of simple carbohydrates. As long as you eat enough protein-rich foods, such as lean meats, fish, and eggs, your body will be able to sustain muscle growth. Also, eating these foods will ensure that you're getting enough dietary fat to keep you healthy.

The following pages present a sample menu incorporating all the major nutrients required to maintain your energy level to keep up with your body's demands as you train and compete. Keep in mind that some of the meals are lower in calories than others. Feel free to experiment, since each person requires a different caloric intake depending on his or her body makeup and level of training. Women and children require fewer calories than the average adult male. It will take you a couple of weeks to determine the right amount and type of food for your body size and demand. To get the exact amounts and the right combination of foods for you, you may want to consult a nutritionist.

BASIC DAILY NUTRITIONAL PLAN

BREAKFAST • 6:30–7:30 A.M.

Option #1
1 cup hot plain oatmeal
20 peanuts or 20 almonds
½ cup strawberries/blueberries or 1 ounce raisins
1 cup of soy milk
1–2 tablespoons honey

Option #2
1–2 poached eggs
1 slice whole-grain toast with 1 teaspoon butter
1 medium baked sweet potato
1 cup fruit salad with ½ cup low-fat cottage cheese

Option #3
Egg omelet (1 whole egg and 2 egg whites)
with bell peppers and mushrooms
4 ounces hash browns or home fries
1 cup mixed broccoli, cauliflower, and carrots

Option #4
2 slices whole-grain French toast
1–2 tablespoons maple syrup
1 cup fruit salad
1 cup low-fat plain yogurt
Coffee or tea with 1 ounce soy milk

Option #5
2 slices whole-grain bread
1 tablespoon peanut butter
1 tablespoon jelly or jam
Coffee or tea with 1 ounce soy milk
¼ cup low-fat milk or 1 cup soymilk
1 medium apple or banana

LUNCH • 10:00–11:30 A.M.

Option #1

4 ounces orange juice

2 ounces of sliced turkey on pumpernickel bread with tomato, lettuce, and 1 teaspoon mayo

unsweetened tea or black coffee

2 teaspoons sugar

2 ounces soy milk

$\frac{1}{2}$ cup blackberries, blueberries, or raspberries

Option #2

4 ounces lentil soup

2 slices rye bread with 1 teaspoon butter

1 cup low-fat plain yogurt

Option #3

Salad greens with 4–5 ounces tuna in water

$\frac{1}{2}$ cup chickpeas

2 tablespoons low-calorie French or Italian dressing

1 small sweet potato or $\frac{1}{2}$ cup cooked bulgur

1 medium orange

1 cup skim milk

unsweetened tea or black coffee

1–2 tablespoons honey

Option #4

4–5 ounce tuna in water

1–2 teaspoons mayo

1 cup romaine lettuce and $\frac{1}{2}$ medium tomato

1 medium apple or $\frac{1}{2}$ medium banana

1–1$\frac{1}{2}$ ounces of semi-soft cheese

SNACKS • 1:30–3:00 P.M. and 9:00–10:00 P.M. (if necessary)

Option #1

1 cup low-fat plain yogurt

$\frac{1}{4}$ cup granola

$\frac{1}{4}$ cup blueberries, strawberries,
or blackberries

Option #2

1 cup skim milk

2 graham crackers

1 small apple or $\frac{1}{2}$ small banana

unsweetened tea or black coffee

1 tablespoon honey

Option #3

25 small pretzel sticks

15 grapes

1 cup low-fat plain yogurt

unsweetened tea or black coffee

1 tablespoon honey

Option #4

1 cup chopped celery
(about 5 medium stalks)

1 tablespoon peanut butter

1 cup low-fat milk or 1 cup soy milk

DINNER • 5:00–6:30 P.M.

Option #1

4 ounces broiled chicken breast

1 plain baked potato plain

1 slice whole-wheat bread

1 cup fresh green beans

Dessert

1 small slice angel food cake without icing
or 6 ounces white wine

1 cup strawberries

Option #2

4 ounces broiled flounder with
1 tablespoon olive oil

$\frac{1}{2}$ cup brown rice

$\frac{1}{2}$ cup broccoli and $\frac{1}{2}$ cup carrots

1 slice whole-wheat bread with
1 tablespoon butter or margarine

Dessert

$\frac{1}{4}$ cantaloupe

8 ounces caffeine-free diet soda

Option #3

8 ounces broiled or grilled ground sirloin burger

$\frac{1}{2}$ cup mixed sautéed mushrooms and onions
in 1 teaspoon olive oil

4 ounces steamed asparagus sprinkled with
1 teaspoon Parmesan cheese

1 medium sweet potato with skin

Dessert

$\frac{1}{4}$ cup fresh cherries

1 glass red wine

unsweetened tea or black coffee

Taking Control of Your Food Intake

- Eat a complete meal that has a combination of protein, carbohydrates, and fat every 2–4 hours.
- Minimize use of refined flour and sugar—for example, sodas, candy, cake, crackers, white bread, and white rice.
- Have your last meal 2–3 hours before bedtime.
- Chew your food slowly and thoroughly.
- Drink water frequently throughout the day, at least eight 8-ounce glasses a day.
- Eat only enough food to feel satiated, not full.
- When dining out, divide your portions and take the extra home with you.
- Put small servings of food on your plate; wait at least 20 minutes before having a second helping.
- Do not keep refined-sugar products such as cookies and crackers in your house—they may be too tempting to avoid.
- Always eat a well-balanced breakfast.
- Eat a variety of foods rather than a few favorite foods.
- Eat at least 2 servings of different-colored fruits and vegetables at each meal.

CONCLUSION

Proper nutrition is essential for optimum performance. This chapter provided the guidelines to follow for finding the most efficient and effective way to eat. As is the case with designing an exercise program, there is an element of art to the science of nutrition. If you find the right combination of foods and the right amounts for you, stick with them until or unless they no longer work. Proper nutrition alone will not turn you in to a champion, but without a proper diet you will always under perform.

As mentioned earlier, if you need more information, consult a knowledgeable and licensed nutritionist and have him or her help you find the right mix for your objective, especially if you have special needs, such as diabetes, high cholesterol, or high blood pressure.

Conclusion

My education and experience have taught me to be flexible but not to be overwhelmed by all the information that's available. I know that the most effective way to succeed is to learn as much as possible about a few things. Having a lot of knowledge about a few essential topics is more beneficial than knowing only a little about everything. Study the weight-training and nutrition principles as you would any other discipline. Absorb the basics and build on that foundation.

Your ultimate success will depend on several parts—your overall conditioning including weight training, your overall nutrition program, and your martial arts training. The right mix of all these elements will determine your level of enjoyment and your level of success. I invite you to be patient, diligent, and savvy about your physical preparation and nutritional choices. I also invite you to be flexible with your program and to have fun with it as well. After all, if you are too competitive and too serious, you can't truly appreciate the beauty of training and gaining.

The material I have covered in this book is not new, but as far as I know, it's the first of its kind for the practitioner of the martial arts. Weight training has been used for years as a way to increase strength and endur-ance. The average practitioner of the martial arts is not any different from other athletes and therefore can use the same techniques to improve his or her performance. The methods and the techniques I have outlined are the most fundamental and, if applied correctly, some of the most effective known to science. The exercises are simple to learn and easy to perform. Once you master proper form, increasing the resistance, the number of sets or the number of reps will be all that is necessary to achieve your desired goal. The routine can remain very basic; you don't need to get fancy to get results. Hard work and dedication are all you need and all that is required to reach the top, but understanding the basic principles provides the foundation to keep you there.

Keep in mind that there are different ways one person can get the same results as someone else. I invite you to experiment with different routines, but your goal should be to find the one method of training that works best for you. I suggest you refer to the book as a guide to refresh your memory every few months. I promise you will find something new every time you go through it. It may be a good idea to read this book in its entirety to get the general idea of the program. Then, break it up into sections and study each one separately as a manual. Rereading certain sections several times may help you get a better sense of the primary meaning. It is crucial to understand the testing procedure. Determining your starting point is essential for a long and healthy relationship with weights. Resist the temptation to progress too quickly because it will increase your chances of overtraining and/or becoming injured.

Above all else, listen to your body. Use common sense and rest when necessary, and get the right medical help if and when it is required. Utilize what you have available to you in terms of equipment, time, and your innate talent. When in doubt, ask an expert or even several experts to get a different perspective. Use this book as a personal guide and perhaps to help others as well. The information outlined in this book should be used only as a guideline for success, not an absolute truth.

Testing Procedures

TESTING FOR MUSCULAR STRENGTH (1RM)

Before you attempt to test your muscular strength, it is important to prepare your body for a maximum level of effort. Warm it up by performing approximately 20 repetitions of the exercise you are getting ready to perform with a low level of resistance—that is, 50 percent of your estimated maximum capacity.

Then, to begin testing your muscular strength, raise the resistance considerably from your warm-up weight, but not quite as high as what you anticipate your maximum would be—that is, increase the weight you just used by 20 percent. Attempt to lift this weight one time (1 rep). After a brief rest period of 30–120 seconds, attempt to lift heavier weight by increasing the resistance as much as is necessary until you reach an amount you cannot lift. The last amount you were able to lift with perfect form and without any help from your spotter is your one-repetition maximum (1RM).

When selecting the appropriate weight to train with, choose 65–90 percent of your 1RM depending on the muscular system you wish to concentrate on—65–80 percent for muscular endurance, 80–95 percent for muscular strength.

TESTING FOR MUSCULAR ENDURANCE (10RM)

Start at a very low level of resistance and attempt to perform 10 repetitions. If you succeed, increase resistance one level or 10 percent after a brief rest period of 60–120 seconds. The last level of resistance at which you are able to complete 10 reps with perfect form is your 10RM.

When selecting the weight to train with, you can go one level lower than your 10RM to work on your muscular endurance or one level above to concentrate on strength building.

In addition to using resistance equipment to test your level of muscular strength or endurance, you can also perform the following tests:

MAXIMUM PUSH-UP TEST

This test is the classic upper-body muscular endurance test, and the average martial arts student is no stranger to it. It is easy to perform, because it requires no equipment and very little space and time.

To perform this test, start in a push-up position with your arms extended, back flat, and hands 20–30 inches apart with your palms flat on the floor and fingers facing the front. Bend your elbows to a ninety-degree angle while lowering your body, then push yourself up. Perform as many push-ups as you can without stopping. If you are not able to complete at least a couple of regular push-ups, you can perform modified push-ups by placing your knees on the floor. On average, men should be able to perform 30–40 push-ups and women, 10–20 push-ups.

ONE-MINUTE MAXIMUM SIT-UP TEST

The one-minute maximum sit-up test will give you a good indication of your abdominal muscle endurance. To perform this test, lie on your back with your feet flat on the floor and your hands supporting the back of your head. Raise your upper body off the floor and up toward your knees by contracting your midsection. Be careful not to pull on your neck. Perform as many of these as you can in one minute. Make sure you are using good form to perform each sit up. Once more, on average, men should be able to perform 40–50 sit-ups and women should be able to perform 20–30 sit-ups.

MAXIMUM PULL-UP/CHIN-UP TEST

The maximum pull-up/chin-up test will give you a good indication of your upper-body muscular strength and/or muscular endurance. This is one of the toughest exercises to perform, because it is very taxing on the large muscle area that is involved. Most people have a hard time being able to pull themselves up even one time. If you are able to pull yourself up at least once without assistance, you can attempt to perform the maximum pull-up/chin-up test. Using an overhand (palms facing away) or an underhand (palms facing you) grip, perform as many pull-ups/chin-ups as you can, making sure you pull your chin over the bar on the way up and extend your arms completely on the way down. Men should be able to perform 10 pull-ups, while women should be able to perform 10 repetitions of 50–60 percent of their body weight using the pull-down or pull-up assist machine. (This piece of equipment is available in most commercial gyms and assists you in doing a pull up by displacing a sufficient amount of your own body weight).

Record the results of the above tests on your copy of the Performance and Progress Log on page 82, so that when you retest every few weeks, you'll be able to see the areas where you've improved and areas that still need work.

PERFORMANCE AND PROGRESS LOG								
Test Dates:								
Lower-Body Strength—One Repetition Maximum (1RM)								
Squat								
Leg press*								
Leg curls								
Upper-Body Strength—One Repetition Maximum (1RM)								
Chest press								
Pull-downs								
Seated rows								
Overhead press								
Lower-Body Strength—Ten Repetition Maximum (10RM)								
Squat								
Leg press*								
Leg curls								
Upper-Body Strength—Ten Repetition Maximum (10RM)								
Chest press								
Pull-downs								
Seated rows								
Overhead press								
Muscular Endurance—Maximum Repetitions								
Pull-ups/Chin-up								
Push-ups								
1-minute sit-ups								

*Leg extensions may be substituted for leg press.

Establishing
Your Objectives

When designing your program, the most important question you have to ask yourself is, *What would I like to accomplish with this training program?* The questions below can help guide you in establishing your goals. Any question where your answer is "yes" should become part of your initial set of objectives.

1. Do you want to improve your overall muscular strength?   Yes   No

2. Do you want to improve your overall muscular endurance?   Yes   No

3. Is it competition related?   Yes   No

   If you answered yes:

   What is your style of martial art?

   What type of competition is it (for example, kata, kickboxing, full and/or no-contact sparring, grappling tournaments)?

   What is the format of competition (elimination 2–3 minutes, multiple 2–3 minute rounds, etc.)?

4. Are you trying to improve punching/blocking effectiveness?   Yes   No

5. Are you trying to improve your stances/kicking power?   Yes   No

6. Are you trying to improve your stamina?   Yes   No

7. Is it injury related: Are you trying to recuperate from an injury
    or strengthen the muscles around a troubled joint?   Yes   No

If you answered yes, indicate the nature and extent of your injury.
(Note: if it is a serious problem you should first consult a physician/physical therapist.)

Once you have established your objectives, select the days you will train and determine how much time you have available for each workout. Be as specific as possible; know the exact days of the week, the exact hour of the day, where you will work out, and for how long. Use the chart below to help you schedule your workouts.

WEEKLY WORKOUT SCHEDULE														
	Monday		Tuesday		Wednesday		Thursday		Friday		Saturday		Sunday	
Duration	AM	PM	AM	PM	AM	PM	AM	PM	AM	PM	AM	PM	AM	PM
30 min														
30–60 min														
60–90 min														
90+ min														

Next, list all the exercises you plan to perform. For each exercise you select, determine the level of resistance (or weight) and the number of reps and sets, and record this information in the tables provided on the following pages.

Consider following the sample workout routines presented in Appendix C. You can change it around later if necessary, but in the beginning, having such a schedule will keep you focused and motivated.

Your initial goals or objectives can be changed over time, but if you change your goals, remember to also change your program. Record all the changes you make since keeping a written record ensures a smooth transition between the different stages of development.

WEIGHT-TRAINING PROGRAM											
DATE											
	1RM	WEIGHT		WEIGHT		WEIGHT		WEIGHT		WEIGHT	
EXERCISE	10RM	REPS	SETS	REPS	SETS	REPS	SETS	REPS	SETS	REPS	SETS

WEIGHT-TRAINING PROGRAM										
DATE										
EXERCISE	1RM 10RM	WEIGHT		WEIGHT		WEIGHT		WEIGHT		WEIGHT
		REPS	SETS	REPS	SETS	REPS	SETS	REPS	SETS	REPS	SETS

WEIGHT-TRAINING PROGRAM

	DATE	1RM	WEIGHT		WEIGHT		WEIGHT		WEIGHT		WEIGHT	
EXERCISE		10RM	REPS	SETS	REPS	SETS	REPS	SETS	REPS	SETS	REPS	SETS

WEIGHT-TRAINING PROGRAM

EXERCISE	DATE 1RM 10RM	WEIGHT		WEIGHT		WEIGHT		WEIGHT		WEIGHT	
		REPS	SETS	REPS	SETS	REPS	SETS	REPS	SETS	REPS	SETS

Sample Training Programs

ONE-WEEK BEGINNER PROGRAM (BASIC MUSCULAR-ENDURANCE TRAINING)	
Monday	
Warm-Up	Jump rope/jumping jacks—10 minutes at an easy pace to loosen up, followed by a 10-minute stretching routine
Lower-body exercises	Basic routine—squats, leg curls, heel raises, ankle flexion, adductor, and abductor
Upper-body exercises	Basic abdominal routine—crunches, upper-body rotations
Weight/resistance level	60–75 percent 1RM or one level below 10RM
Reps	12–20 reps or 30–60 second intervals
Sets	1–2 sets
Rest between sets	30–90 seconds
Tuesday	

If you feel extremely sore or fatigued after Monday's workout, you may skip the weights and concentrate on martial arts training. If you feel up to the task, perform the following routine:

Warm-Up	Same as Monday
Lower-body exercises	None—recovery day
Upper-body exercises	Basic back routine—pull-ups (regular grip), seated rows (alternative-inverted grip pull-ups), back extensions. Basic shoulder routine—overhead presses, lateral raises; biceps curls, triceps push-downs

Weight/resistance level	Same as Monday
Reps	Same as Monday
Sets	Same as Monday
Rest between sets	Same as Monday

Wednesday

Rest day if you weight trained Monday and Tuesday. No weight training and very little or no karate training.

Thursday

Repeat Monday's workout.

Friday

Repeat Tuesday's workout.

Saturday

Complete rest day. Absolutely no training of any kind. Limit all other activity levels as well.

Sunday

Take this day off if you need more time to recover. Do not forget this is your first week of training. If you do too much too soon, you will stop yourself before you get a chance to start. If you feel well rested after Saturday's day off, complete the following routine:

Warm-Up	5–10 minutes
Lower-body exercises	Basic lower-body routine plus leg extensions
Upper-body exercises	Basic back routine, chest press, crunches
Weight/resistance level	Same as Monday
Reps	Same as Monday
Sets	Same as Monday
Rest between sets	Same as Monday

If you do not have the luxury of time or you only have two or three days a week to devote to weight training, you may combine the Monday and Tuesday workouts into a one-day workout. This means you have to keep the number of sets at one per exercise in order to complete each routine and still be productive. There is really not much difference between the two alternatives.

ONE-WEEK INTERMEDIATE PROGRAM

Monday

Warm-Up	Jump rope/jumping jacks—10 minutes, stretching routine—10 minutes
Lower-body exercises	Basic routine, lunges or leg extensions
Upper-body exercises	Basic abdominal, upper-body rotations or bicycle kicks
Weight/resistance level	70–85 percent 1RM or 10RM
Reps	8–12 reps or 30–45 second intervals
Sets	2–4 sets
Rest between sets	60–90 seconds

Tuesday

If you feel extremely sore or fatigued after Monday's workout, skip the weights and concentrate on karate training. If you feel up to the task, perform the following routine:

Warm-Up	Same as Monday
Lower-body exercises	None—recovery day
Upper-body exercises	Basic back routine, basic shoulder routine, bent-over raises, biceps curls, triceps push-downs
Weight/resistance level	Same as Monday
Reps	Same as Monday
Sets	Same as Monday
Rest between sets	Same as Monday

Wednesday

If you weight trained on Monday and Tuesday—rest day; no weight training and little or no karate training. If you took Tuesday off, do Tuesday's workout.

Thursday

Repeat Monday's workout unless you need another day off after training on Wednesday.

Friday

Repeat Tuesday's workout, or if you took Thursday off, do Monday's workout.

Saturday	

Complete rest day, or repeat Tuesday's workout if you didn't complete it the second time this week.

Sunday	

Take this day off if you need it. If you feel good, do the following routine:

Warm-Up	5–10 minutes
Lower-body exercises	Basic lower body routine
Upper-body exercises	Basic back routine, chest press, crunches
Weight/resistance level	55–70 percent 1RM
Reps	As many as you can even if it is more than 20 reps
Sets	1–2 sets
Rest between sets	Same amount of time it takes you to complete the set, take more time if needed

If you are short on time, it's enough to keep the workouts at basic-training level without adding more exercises. Instead, alternate between similar exercises to keep it interesting. The number of sets does not have to be above 3. You can also combine the workouts as I recommended for the basic stage if you do not have a full week at your disposal. It is the intensity of work that is the most important variable, and as long as you max-out during each set, you will improve with time. The number of repetitions should be no more than 12 at the end of this period unless otherwise instructed (see Sunday workout).

Now you are ready for some real work. Do not forget to take a week off before retesting yourself and stepping up to a new level of training.

ONE-WEEK ADVANCED PROGRAM (STRENGTH BUILDING)	
Monday	
Warm-Up	Jump rope/jumping jacks—10 minutes, stretching routine—10 minutes
Lower-body exercises	Basic routine, lunges or leg extensions
Upper-body exercises	Basic abdominal, upper-body rotations and bicycle kicks
Weight/resistance level	80–95 percent 1RM
Reps	3–8 reps or 15–30 second intervals
Sets	2–4 sets
Rest between sets	At least two minutes

Tuesday	
Rest day.	

Wednesday	
Warm-Up	Same as Monday
Lower-body exercises	None—recovery day
Upper-body exercises	Basic back routine, basic shoulder routine, bent-over raises; biceps curls, triceps push-downs
Weight/resistance level	Same as Monday
Reps	Same as Monday
Sets	Same as Monday
Rest between sets	Same as Monday

Thursday	
Day off or repeat Monday's workout if you feel up to it.	

Friday	
Repeat Monday's workout if you took Thursday off, or rest day.	

Saturday	
Complete rest day or Wednesday's workout if you took Friday off.	

Sunday	
Wednesday's workout if you rested on Saturday or a day off.	

If you feel this new level of intensity is too much to handle for the entire week, you can lower the intensity for the second workout of the week. As long as you include a strength-building workout and an endurance-building workout for each body part during the week, you will be able to reap the benefits of your labor.

ONE-WEEK MAINTENANCE PROGRAM	
Monday	
Warm-Up	Jump rope/jumping jacks—10 minutes; stretching routine—10 minutes
Lower-body exercises	Basic routine
Upper-body exercises	Basic abdominal, upper-body rotations and bicycle kicks
Weight/resistance level	75–90 percent 1RM or 10RM

Reps	6–12 reps or 20–45 second intervals
Sets	2–3 sets
Rest between sets	60–120 seconds

Tuesday

Rest day. Absolutely no weight training and preferably no karate training.

Wednesday

Warm-Up	Same as Monday
Lower-body exercises	None—recovery day
Upper-body exercises	Basic back routine, basic shoulder routine, biceps curls, triceps push-downs
Weight/resistance level	Same as Monday
Reps	Same as Monday
Sets	Same as Monday
Rest between sets	Same as Monday

Thursday

Same as Tuesday.

Friday

Rest day or do the following routine:

Warm-Up	Jump rope/jumping jacks—10 minutes; stretching routine—10 minutes
Lower-body exercises	Basic routine
Upper-body exercises	Basic abdominal, basic back, basic shoulder, biceps curls, triceps push-downs
Weight/resistance level	70–80 percent 1RM or 10RM
Reps	10–15 reps or 30–60 second intervals
Sets	2–3 sets
Rest between sets	60–120 seconds

Saturday

Rest day or Friday's workout if you decided to take Friday off.

Sunday

Complete rest if possible.

Index

Note: **Bolded** page numbers indicate exercise descriptions.

Y

About the Author

Mikhail Krupnik discovered the art of self-defense as a young boy in the late 1970s. He became fascinated with the likes of Bruce Lee and Chuck Norris, and joined his neighborhood karate school. From ages fifteen to eighteen, Krupnik dominated the local tournament circuit and won a number of open and AAU-sponsored competitions, including three state titles and one national title. Then, competing as an adult in 1985, Krupnik's performance at the Maccabiah Games earned him a gold medal. This was the highlight of his competitive career, which was cut short due to injuries.

Yearning for new challenges, Krupnik started weight training and running in addition to his karate practice. At age twenty-two, he began competing in races and triathlons to satisfy his competitive nature. In nine years of competition, he successfully completed approximately ninety races, including more than fifty triathlons, and won dozens of age-group awards.

As his competitive career was nearing the end, his professional career was just beginning. After earning his master's degree from Queens College, Krupnik began teaching fitness and weight training courses at John Jay College of Criminal Justice in New York City, where he also assumed the duties of supervising exercise professional for the fitness center. Krupnik has also supervised exercise prescription classes at New York University and has lectured for the Health and Hospitals Corporation on the subject of health and fitness. He also supervised a New York City female firefighter cadet program.

Presently, Krupnik owns and operates a martial arts and personal training studio in Port Washington, New York. He continues to conduct lectures and workshops on weight training for the martial arts.

www.ingramcontent.com/pod-product-compliance
Lightning Source LLC
Jackson TN
JSHW011405130125
77033JS00023B/861